RECENT RESULTS OF
CANCER TREATMENT IN JAPAN

GANN Monograph on Cancer Research

The series of GANN Monograph on Cancer Research was initiated in 1966 by the late Dr. Tomizo Yoshida (1903–73) for the purpose of publishing proceedings of international conferences and symposia on cancer and allied research fields, and papers on specific subjects of importance in cancer research.

The decision to publish a monograph is made by the Editorial Board of the Japanese Cancer Association, with the final approval of the Board of Directors. It is hoped that the series will serve as an important source of information in cancer research.

Japanese Cancer Association

The publication of this monograph owes much to the financial support given by the late Professor Kazushige Higuchi of Jikei University.

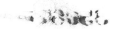

JAPANESE CANCER ASSOCIATION

GANN Monograph on Cancer Research No. 22

RECENT RESULTS OF CANCER TREATMENT IN JAPAN

TAMAKI KAJITANI

Edited by YOSHIYUKI KOYAMA

YOICHIRO UMEGAKI

JAPAN SCIENTIFIC SOCIETIES PRESS, Tokyo
UNIVERSITY PARK PRESS, Baltimore

Published jointly by
JAPAN SCIENTIFIC SOCIETIES PRESS
Tokyo
and
UNIVERSITY PARK PRESS
Baltimore

ISBN 0-8391-1415-X
Library of Congress Catalogue Card No. 79-51265

PREFACE

Surgical treatment of cancer in Japan was in its infancy in the 1940's but made a remarkable advance in the 1950's. The standard and extended radical operation techniques for cancer of various organs became established in the 1950's. In spite of extended surgical treatment, direct mortality from surgery decreased markedly and surgery became quite a safe method of treatment. This is due not only to the progress in anesthesia and surgical techniques but also to the enormous advances in medical science made after World War II.

In the field of radiotherapy, the progress in high-energy radiation apparatus (telecobalt, linear accelerator, beratron, *etc.*) greatly contributed to the improvement in treatment results. Much effort has been concentrated, not only on the improvement in survival rate but also on the status of patients in their social lives by the preservation of vital functions. As a result of these improvements, radiotherapy is increasingly being selected as the first choice of treatment of cancer in certain sites.

Recently, high LFT radiations and heavy ions were introduced but clinical experience with these modalities is so limited that the results could not be included in this volume. Evaluation of the results will probably be possible in the next ten years.

In the field of cancer chemotherapy, Nitromin (nitrogen mustard N-oxide) began to be used clinically in 1950 in Japan and discovery of mitomycin-C has widely promoted cancer chemotherapy. After the introduction of another new antibiotic, bleomycin, in 1966, the correlation of the histological type of tumor with the effectiveness of each chemotherapeutic was observed.

Treatment with multiple combinations of chemotherapeutics was started in 1962, and this method of treatment began to be used extensively in 1965 and 1966 when cyclophosphamide and 5-fluorouracil, respectively, became available in Japan. At present, multidrug combination therapy is being carried out with various agents, including alkylating agents, antimetabolites, anticancer antibiotics and plant products. The duration of treatment is also being extended.

Recent chemotherapy of cancer is showing notable results, and 5-year sruvival, although low in number, is found in some of the advanced tumors in which surgery was not indicated. The period for 50% survival from the beginning of treatment is also increasing annually. It is still too early to present 5-year survival results in this monograph but it is hoped that they will be published in the nerar future.

During the 1960's, early detection of cancer, which was the main cause of improvement in the treatment results of cancer, was made easier by the advance of diagnostics and mass screening of the population. In addition to individual studies on surgery, radiotherapy and chemotherapy, the multidisciplinary intensive treatment of cancer by combined use has been developed. Consequently, new methods of cancer treatment were successively established, and the therapeutic results are now available for cancer of many organs.

In this volume of the GANN Monograph on Cancer Research, more than 15 kinds of cancer, some prevalent in Japan and some rare but that seem specific in Japan, have been highlighted, and the methods as well as the results of treatment, mainly in the 1960's have been described. For the evaluation of treatment results, institutions which hav experience with a large number of cases for each of the organs, have been selected. In the case of breast, lung, stomach, and uterine cancer, many institutions in Japan have cooperated in the clinical study and their accumulated results have been published. Some of the articles are on the comparative evaluation of results with historical controls obtained before the 1960's, and there are also articles on the treatment of cancer which showed a marked improvement in the 1970's.

The last article in this volume is on " Cancer Statistics in Japan and Osaka," based on the results of a research group for population-based cancer registration. This article is of the statistics on cancer incidence in six prefectures in Japan, and summarizes cancers of particular organs prevalent in Japan, states of the treatment, and 5-year survival rates.

This volume of GANN Monograph on Cancer Research gives representative results of cancer treatment in Japan during the 1960's, and it is believed that this volume will offer important material for the study of therapeutic methods of cancer in the future. We will be pleased if this volume proves to be a valuable milestone in the evaluation of the improvement in cancer treatment and its results in 10 or 20 years.

December 1978

Tamaki KAJITANI
Yoshiyuki KOYAMA
Yoichiro UMEGAKI

CONTENTS

viii

CANCER OF THE ORAL CAVITY

Chisato Taketa, Yoichiro Umegaki, Shizumi Matsuura,
Isamu Ono, Satoshi Ebihara, and Kunio Washizu

Division of Head and Neck, Department of Radiation Therapy,
*National Cancer Center Hospital**

Oral carcinoma cases consisted of 2.8% of all malignant diseases at the National Cancer Center, 21% of head and neck cancer, and 29% of cancer of the upper aero-digestive tract. A total of 376 cases of carcinoma of the oral cavity were treated during the 10 years from 1962 to 1971 and were followed up for 5 years or until death.

This study analyzes 281 previously untreated cases of squamous cell carcinoma in terms of treatment and results. There were 194 cases of carcinoma of the tongue, 29 cases of floor of the mouth, 21 cases of gingiva, 17 cases of buccal mucosa, 15 cases of hard palate, and 5 cases of carcinoma of the lip. Radiation therapy was performed on the majority of cases whereas persistent or recurrent lesions underwent operation. Relative survival rate for all cases was 72%, for lip 99%, for floor of mouth 76%, buccal mucosa 75%, hard palate 69%, tongue 68%, and for gingiva 66%. Relative survival rate for Stage I was 78%, Stage II 76%, Stage III 55%, and for Stage IV 41%.

Carcinoma of the tongue appears to be best controlled by interstitial radium therapy, and radium implant or electron beam irradiation is effective for localized or superficial lesions of the lip or buccal mucosa. Surgery is indicated for cancer of the oral floor, gingiva, and palate. The introduction of reconstructive surgery widened the indication of operation and also the sphere of radical therapy.

The incidence of carcinoma of the oral cavity in Japan has not been exactly defined. Oral carcinoma cases accounted for 2.8% of all malignant diseases at the National Cancer Center Hospital, Tokyo; 21% of head and neck cancer, and 29% of cancer of the upper respiratory and digestive tract (7).

Definition of the Series

A total of 376 cases of carcinoma of the oral cavity were treated at the National Cancer Center Hospital during the 10-year period from 1962 to 1971 and were followed-up for 5 years or until death. Cases excluded from this survey consisted of 72 cases which had received previous treatment at other institutions and 23 cases of adenocarcinoma. This study analyzes 281 previously untreated cases of squamous cell carcinoma in terms of treatment and results (Table I).

* Tsukiji 5-1-1, Chuo-ku, Tokyo 104, Japan (竹田千里, 梅垣洋一郎, 松浦 鎮, 小野 勇, 海老原 敏, 鷲津邦雄).

TABLE I. Classification of Treated Patients by Region and Stage

Region	Stage				Total
	I	II	III	IV	
Tongue	56	60	28	50	194
Floor of mouth	3	7	3	16	29
Gingiva	5	3	4	9	21
Buccal mucosa	1	5	3	8	17
Hard palate	9	3	2	1	15
Lip	2	1		2	5
Total number	76	79	40	86	281

Therapeutic Methods

Primarily we applied radiation therapy in the majority of cases for as long as they displayed a response. When a lesion could not be controlled by this method or when a recurrence was found surgical therapy was applied. External irradiation was given by a 6 MeV Linac X-ray and/or Betatron electron-beam irradiation. Electron beam therapy was also employed for intracavitary irradiation, while radium needles were used for interstitial irradiation (1, 2, 5, 8, 9).

Details of the primary treatment are shown in Table II. Out of a total of 281 cases only 63 underwent surgery as the first treatment; however, as surgery was applied in uncontrollable or recurrent cases, a total of 112 cases underwent operation.

During the period of the study, we discovered that, apart from tongue and lip cases, carcinoma of the oral cavity is better controlled by surgery, and this method came to be the predominant therapeutic approach. Indications for operation have increased markedly since the introduction of reconstructive surgery (3, 4, 6, 12) in 1970. When metastatic lymph nodes were detected, radical neck dissection was generally performed—in 38 cases as part of the primary treatment, and in another 38 cases to control late metastasis.

TABLE II. Methods of Primary Treatment

Region	Treatment					Total number
	Radium implant	Intracavitary electron	External irradiation	Chemotherapy +irradiation	Surgery	
Tongue	110	35	9	2	38	194
Floor of mouth	10	2	5	1	11	29
Gingiva	4	2	5	2	8	21
Buccal mucosa	6	0	8	1	2	17
Hard palate	1	6	3	1	4	15
Lip	2	0	3	0	0	5
Total number	133	45	33	7	63	281

Therapeutic Results

1. Carcinoma of the tongue

The age and sex distribution of cases shown in Fig. 1 indicates a peak at 60 years of age and a male-to-female ratio of 2 : 1. The primary therapeutic method in this group was interstitial radium therapy. Intracavitary electron beam therapy was applied only to superficial lesions 2 cm or less in diameter, while external irradiation was often applied as palliative treatment in extensive cases (*11*).

Surgery was selected as the primary therapy in 38 cases in the following two categories (*11*):

i) Composite operation in extensive cases in which invasion extended beyond the tongue (*12*).

ii) Local excision of small superficial lesions.

Therapeutic methods and results are summarized in Tables III and IV. Of 156

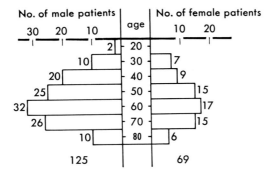

Fig. 1.   Age and sex distribution of the tongue cancer cases

TABLE III.   Results of Treatment of Tongue Carcinoma

Treatment	No. of cases	No. of 5-year survivors	5-Year survival rate (%)
Radium implant	110	72	65.4
Intracavitary electron	35	26	74.2
External irradiation	9	2	22.2
Chemotherapy + irradiation	2	0	0
Surgery	38	14	36.8
Total number	194	114	58.7

TABLE IV.   Results of Surgery for Carcinoma of the Tongue

	No. of caess	No. of 5-year survivors	5-Year survival rate (%)
Local excision	24	12	50.0
Composite operation	14	2	14.2
Hemiglossectomy	2	1	
Total glossectomy	12	1	
Total number	38	14	36.8

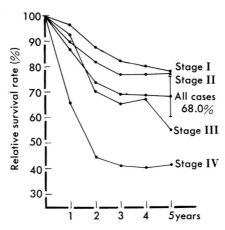

FIG. 2.   Relative survival curves for the 194 cases of tongue cancer

cases which received radiation therapy, 63 cases (40.4%) survived for 5 years or more without recurrence. In 33 cases recurrence was observed at the primary site and at the neck lymph nodes in 39, totalling 72 cases. Death due to insufficiently effective primary irradiation occurred in 16 cases, and 5 other cases died of other diseases within 5 years.

Primary site recurrence was treated by total glossectomy in 7 cases and hemi-glossectomy in 21, and 13 of these 28 cases were well-controlled. In 2 cases of recurrence in which the primary therapy had been intracavitary electron beam, control was established by means of re-irradiation with radium. However, re-irradiation was not effective in other cases.

Of 39 recurrence cases with lymph node metastasis to the neck, 34 underwent radical neck dissection, and cancer was controlled in 21 of these. Radiation was performed in 4 cases, but without success.

In terms of therapeutic efficacy surgery appeared to be the most significant in recurrent cases of tongue cancer. Survival curves for each stage are shown in Fig. 2.

2.   Carcinoma of the floor of the mouth

Overall 5-year survival figures according to primary therapy are shown in Table V, and Table VI provides a breakdown of irradiation therapy figures. In 18 cases which received radiation therapy, death from failure of the primary therapy was seen in 1 case, recurrence at the primary site was observed in 7 cases, metastasis to neck lymph nodes in 2, while 2 cases each died of lung metastasis and primary cancer of

TABLE V.   Results of Treament of Carcinoma of Floor of the Mouth

	No. of cases	No. of 5-year survivors	5-Year survival rate (%)
Surgery	11	10	90.0
Radiation therapy	18	9[a]	50.0
Total number	29	19	65.5

[a] Five cases salvaged by secondary operation included.

TABLE VI. Results of Radiation Therapy for Carcinoma of Floor of the Mouth

	No. of cases	No. of 5-year survivors	5-Year survival rate (%)
Radium implant	10	6	60.0
Intracavitary electron	5	2	40.0
External irradiation	3	1	33.3
Total number	18	9[a]	50.0

[a] Five cases required salvage by surgical intervention.

other organs. No recurrence was seen in 4 cases (22.2%). The 7 cases which exhibited recurrence at the primary site underwent surgery, and 4 of these were controlled and the remaining 3 succumbed to lung metastasis.

In general, radiation therapy appears to have only a limited effect in preventing recurrence at the primary site, and metastasis to the neck and to other organs is noted frequently. Local control by radium therapy appears to be relatively good, although late necrosis of the mandible is sometimes seen.

Of 11 surgically treated cases, there was not a single instance of local recurrence but one death occurred due to metastasis to the neck lymph nodes.

3. Carcinoma of the gingiva

Table VII shows the 5-year survivals according to the primary therapeutic method. Of 13 radiation therapy cases, 5 died from failure of the primary treatment and there were 6 cases of recurrence, as compared to only 2 cases of survival without recurrence (15.4%). In 5 cases of primary site recurrence in which salvage operations were performed, 2 were well-controlled. One case which received cryotherapy was also well-controlled. In all, 5 cases were well-controlled and 8 died.

On the other hand, of 8 patients who received surgery as the primary therapy 7 are surviving after more than 5 years, which indicates the better efficacy of surgical therapy in carcinoma of the gingiva, which is particularly true since the introduction of reconstruction surgery.

TABLE VII. Results of Therapy for Carcinoma of Gingiva

Primary treatment	No. of cases	No. of 5-year survivors	5-Year survival rate (%)
Surgery	8	7	87.5
Radiation therapy	13	5[a]	38.5
Total number	21	12	57.1

[a] Two cases were secondarily controlled by surgery, and one by cryotherapy.

4. Carcinoma of the buccal mucosa

Five-year survival figures are shown in Table VIII. Of the 15 cases receiving radiation therapy, the primary lesion was controlled by irradiation in 5 cases (33.3%) only, and the remaining 10 cases exhibited local recurrence. In 4 cases of salvage operation with simultaneous reconstruction, good control was achieved in 3 cases. One case

TABLE VIII. Results of Treatment of Carcinoma of the Buccal Mucosa

Primary treatment	No. of cases	No. of 5-year survivors	5-Year survival rate (%)
Surgery	2	1	50.0
Radiation therapy	15[a]	8[b]	53.3
Total number	17	9	52.9

[a] Combined with radical neck dissection in 5 cases.
[b] Three cases which developed local recurrence were controlled by surgery.

died of metastasis to the neck, and another due to unknown causes. Surgery was adopted as the primary therapeutic approach in only 2 cases in which the tumor was extensive. Our results suggest that superficial cancer of the buccal mucosa be treated by irradiation and penetrating lesions by composite operation combined with reconstruction.

5. Carcinoma of the hard palate

The 5-year survival figures shown in Table IX indicate that all 4 patients who underwent surgery as the primary therapy are surviving after 5 years or more, while only 2 cases (18.2%) were controlled by irradiation alone.

TABLE IX. Results of Therapy for Carcinoma of the Hard Palate

Primary treatment	No. of cases	No. of 5-year survivors	5-Year survival rate (%)
Surgery	4	4	100.0
Radiation therapy	11	5[a]	45.5
Total number	15	9	60.0

[a] Three cases which developed local recurrence were controlled by surgery.

6. Carcinoma of the lip

Out of 5 cases receiving irradiation therapy, 4 were controlled by irradiation only. The single ease of recurrence underwent surgery but did not survive 5 years.

DISCUSSION AND CONCLUSIONS

Radiation and/or surgical therapy was performed in 281 cases of squamous cell carcinoma of the oral cavity and observations were made for 5 years or more in surviving cases. Relative survival rates for all cases in each stage are shown in Fig. 3, and Fig. 4 shows the survival curves for each region. Carcinoma of the tongue appears to be best controlled by interstitial radium therapy, and radium implant or electron beam irradiation is effective for localized or superficial lesions of the lip or buccal mucosa. Surgery is indicated for cancer of the oral floor, gingiva, and palate. The introduction of reconstruction surgery in 1970 widened the indications of operation and also the sphere of radical therapy (*12*).

Although chemotherapy (*10*) and cryotherapy are in widespread use at present they were seldom employed in this series. These modalities appear promising in the

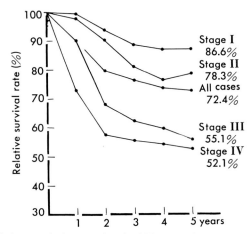

FIG. 3.   Relative survival curves for the 281 cases of carcinoma of the mouth

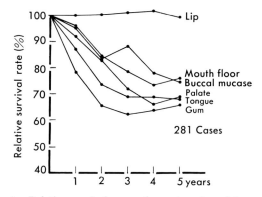

FIG. 4.   Relative survival curves for each region of the mo. th

reduction of irradiation dosage therapy limiting or eliminating side-effects, and also in avoiding disfiguration and dysfunction caused by resection of a wide area.

Acknowledgment

This study was supported in part by a Grant-in-Aid for Cancer Research from the Ministry of Health and Welfare.

REFERENCES

1.   Ash, C. L. Oral cancer: A twenty-five year study. *Am. J. Roentgenol. Radium Ther. Nucl. Med.*, **86**, 417–430 (1962).

2.   Frazell, E. L. and Lucas J. C. Cancer of the tongue. Report of the management of 1,554 patients. *Cancer*, **15**, 1085–1099 (1962).

3.   Fujino, T. Contribution of the axial and perforator vasculature to circulation in flaps. *Plast. Reconstr. Surg.*, **39**, 125–137 (1967).

4.   Hoopes, J. E. and Edgerston, M. T. Immediate forehead flap repair in resection for oropharyngeal cancer. *Am. J. Surg.*, **112**, 526–533 (1966).

5.   Martin, H. E. The history of lingual cancer. *Am. J. Surg.*, **98**, 703–716 (1940).

6. McGregor, I. A. and Jackson, I. T. The extended role of the delto-pectoral flap. *Br. J. Plast. Surg.*, **23**, 173–185 (1970).

7. Nakahara, W. and Taketa, C. "Atlas of Head and Neck Cancer," Nakayama Shoten, Tokyo (1975) (in Japanese).

8. Quimby, E. H. "Physical Foundation of Radiology," Paul B. Hoeber Inc. (1952).

9. Paterson, R. "The Treatment of Malignant Disease by Radiotherapy," Edward Arnold Ltd., London (1963).

10. Taketa, C., Shimosato, Y., Nagano, A., Washizu, K., Matsuura, S., Ono, I., and Ebihara, S. Effects of bleomycin for epidermoid carcinoma of head and neck. *Nippon Gan Chiryo Gakkaishi (J. Japan. Soc. Cancer Ther.)*, **1**, 41–53 (1971) (in Japanese).

11. Taketa, C. and Washizu, K. Carcinoma of the tongue. *Nippon Gan Chiryo Gakkaishi (J. Japan. Soc. Cancer Ther.)*, **20**, 301–310 (1974) (in Japanese).

12. Taketa, C., Ono, I., Ebihara, S., Suzuki, K., and Washizu, K. Surgical treatment of head and neck carcinomas simultaneously combined with reconstruction. *Rinsho Jibika (Pract. Otol., Kyoto)*, **69**, 465–480 (1976) (in Japanese).

CANCER OF THE MAXILLARY SINUS

Chisato Taketa, Yoichiro Umegaki, Shizumi Matsuura,
Isamu Ono, Satoshi Ebihara, and Kunio Washizu

Division of Head and Neck, Department of Radiation Therapy,
*National Cancer Center Hospital**

1. One hundred and fifty-five previously untreated patients with squamous cell carcinoma of the maxillary sinus are presented. A comparison between the treatment results of arterial chemotherapy combined and not combined was attempted. The relative 5-year survival rate of the total series was 52.7%. Observed survival rate was 48%.

2. Some advantages of arterial chemotherapy combined with radiation were demonstrated. Survival was considerably improved by this treatment, especially in advanced cases. The most distinct advantage of this arterial chemotherapy combined treatment was a decrease in the number of patients who needed aggressive surgery, hence the rehabilitation of the patients was markedly improved.

3. Recent experience indicated that by combination of arterial chemotherapy, the dose of radiation can be decreased to 4,000 rad. By this new trial of treatment, complications such as damage of the eye, bone necrosis, and intracranial complications have hardly been observed and the result of the treatment will be at least the same as that of this series.

In the last 10 years, the treatment policy for carcinoma of the maxillary sinus has changed considerably in our country. The change was observed as follows: 1) Combined arterial infusion chemotherapy with radiation therapy has been generally accepted to be useful in improving the result of the treatment. 2) A strong tendency to lessen the dose of radiation has been prevalent. 3) The number of cases in which aggressive surgery was performed, like total maxillectomy, has dramatically decreased.

However, sufficient analysis of this treatment modality, especially of the end result of the treatment, has not yet been done. Therefore, the main purpose of the present communication is to record the benefits of treatment by comparison with treatment by uncombined arterial chemotherapy.

Definition of the Series

During 1962 to 1971, 259 patients with cancer of the nasal cavity, paranasal sinuses, and other adjoining structures visited the National Cancer Center Hospital, Tokyo. Primary sites and histopathology of the cases are shown in Table I. They comprised approximately 16% of all patients with head-and-neck malignancies, and 2% of all

---

* Tsukiji 5-1-1, Chuo-ku, Tokyo 104, Japan (竹田千里, 梅垣洋一郎, 松浦 鎮, 小野 勇, 海老原 敏, 鷲津邦雄).

C. TAKETA ET AL.

TABLE I. Anatomic Site and Histopathology of Total Series

		Squamous carcinoma	Adeno carcinoma	Adenoid cystic carcinoma	Melanoma	Malignant lymphoma	Other malig. or hist. unavailable	Total number
Primary cases	Maxillary sinus	155	4	6			1	166
	Nasal cavity	2			2	1	3	8
	Frontal sinus	2						2
	Not clear		1			2	4	7
Secondary cases	Maxillary sinus	52	2	2			7	63
	Nasal cavity	2					2	4
	Frontal sinus	2						2
	Not clear	1				4	2	7
	Total	216	7	8	2	7	19	259

(1962–1971, National Cancer Center Hospital, Tokyo).

human cancer cases who visited and were registered during the same period in our hospital. This incidence does not demonstrate the true incidence for human cancers in our country, because the patients with head-and-neck malignancies have a tendency to be referred to a central hospital like the Cancer Institute Hospital or University Hospitals. The true incidence of the cancer of nasal cavity and paranasal sinus cancer is quite difficult to determine, but it can be estimated to be less than 1% of all human cancers. Nevertheless, the incidence of carcinoma of the maxillary sinus may be higher than that in Europe and U.S.A. (1, 5, 6, 11).

In this study, analysis of the patients was limited to 155 patients who had not been treated before coming to our clinic and histologically diagnosed as squamous cell carcinoma of the maxillary sinus. However, some cases of carcinoma of the ethmoid sinus might be included because it was often difficult to differentiate them from carcinoma of the maxillary sinus. Patients with malignant minor salivary gland tumors, malignant lymphoma, melanoma, and those for whom no pathological diagnosis was available were excluded, because the treatment of these malignancies and their prognoses are quite different from those of squamous cell carcinoma of the maxillary sinus.

Distribution of Age and Sex

The average age of the patients in the entire series was 55 years. The male to female ratio was 2:1. This age and sex distribution was in agreement with other studies (1, 11).

Methods and Treatment

The patients were divided into 2 groups by treatment methods. One was treated by combined arterial infusion and chemotherapy (AI series), the other was not combined with arterial infusion (no-AI series). The chemotherapeutic agent was administered by placing a Teflon catheter in the external carotid artery. The superficial temporal artery was the usual route of insertion of the catheter. The catheter was fixed just at the position where facial artery distribution was stained by the injection of Patent Blue.

Patients had simultaneous drainage by making a large opening on the anterior wall of the maxillary sinus. This drainage opening must be large enough to be able to observe the whole aspect of the sinus. A nasal-antral window was usually made by removing lateral structures of the nasal cavity.

The tumor dose of radiation ranged from 6,000 to 8,000 rad in most of the no-AI series and from 4,000 to 6,000 rad in most of the AI series. Intracavitary irradiation was often combined after surgery in the no-AI series.

As a chemotherapeutic agent, 5-fluorouracil was used in most of the cases during the years of this series' treatment. The dose was 250 mg daily, the total dose ranging from 2,500 to 5,000 mg given by one-shot injection manually or sometimes given continuously by a pump.

Of all the procedures, it is most important to keep the maxillary sinus under good observation and maintain the sinus and its adjoining structures clear by aspirating and removing necroric tissue every day so that, usually, at the end of the combined treatment, most of the structures around the maxillary sinus except the orbit and the palate have already been removed before final surgery is performed.

As a final treatment, surgery was performed. The main purpose of this procedure was to remove necrotic tissue and to certify the effect of the treatment histologically. Therefore, this surgical removal was not so aggressive, usually the orbit and palate were preserved as far as possible. Total maxillectomy was seldom performed, especially in the AI series.

Classification of Cases

The TNM classification of maxillary cancer has not been agreed upon by the UICC. The cases in our clinic have been classified retrospectively according to our own TNM classification, as shown in Table II.

Results of Treatment

Results of treatment of the total series and each classification are shown in Fig. 1. This survival curve was calculated by the relative survival according to the proposal of the International Symposium on End Results of Cancer Therapy (Norway, 1963).

In the total series from 1962 to 1971, a relative survival of 52.7% was obtained. The observed 5-year survival rate was 48%. Out of 155 patients, 83 could not be controlled. Causes of failure were persistent or recurrent carcinoma (67 cases), intercurrent disease (8 cases), carcinoma of double primary (4 cases), unknown disease (1 case), and lost to follow-up (3 cases).

The vast majority of persistent or recurrent carcinoma were found in the primary site as reported in other studies (6, 7). This is the reason why control of the primary lesion is most important for obtaining a better result.

Cervical node metastases were not common in carcinoma of the maxillary sinus (3, 5, 7). In this series, only 12 cases (7.7%)had clinically positive nodes before treatment. Prognosis of the patients with cervical node involvement is generally considered

TABLE II.   Classification of Carcinoma of the Maxillary Sinus in
National Cancer Center Hospital, Tokyo

T_{1s}		Pre-invasive carcinoma (carcinoma *in situ*)
T_1		Tumor limited to the maxillary sinus without any evidence of bone involvement
T_2		Destruction of bony wall without or slight involvement of surrounding tissue (Involvement of the nasal cavity and slight invasion of the ethmoid sinus included in this criterion)
T_3		Marked invasion to the surrounding tissue
T_{3a}	1)	Destruction of bone in more than two directions
	2)	Destruction of posterior wall or the body of zygomatic bone
	3)	Swelling of floor of the nasal cavity or alveolar process or the hard palate
	4)	marked invasion to ethmoid sinus or orbit
T_{3b}	1)	Destruction of pterigoid process or trismus
	2)	Swelling of inner canthus of the eye or zygomatic area
	3)	Objective hypoesthesia of skin of the cheek or the hard palate
	4)	Limited movement of the orbit
T_4		Advanced case which is most difficult to control
	1)	Disturbance of eyesight or complete fixation of the orbit
	2)	Marked swelling of temporal fossa and its adjoining soft tissue
	3)	Invasion and penetration to the skin
	4)	Involvement of the mesopharynx or nasopharynx or parapharyngeal space
	5)	Involvement of the sphenoid sinus or frontal sinus Destruction of the skull base or any evidence of intracranial involvement

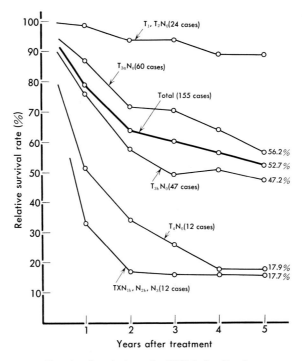

FIG. 1.   Survival rate by TNM classification

to be poor (*1*). It proved to be true in our series. Out of 12 patients, only 2 were controlled more than 5 years. However, metastases of these 2 patients were treated by radiation therapy and histological diagnosis of node involvement was not available.

The TNM classification by our own criteria corresponded fairly well with survivals. However, the difference between T_{3a} and T_{3b} was not so definite as expected.

The observed 5-year survival rate of the AI series and no-AI series were 59.5% and 46.7%, respectively. Slight superiority of the AI series was observed but this difference was not statistically significant. However, it must be borne in mind that in the AI series there were more advanced cases than in the no-AI series. Comparison of the results of the treatment between the AI series and no-AI series in advanced cases (T_{3b} and T_4) revealed a distinct difference (Fig. 2). This difference was also too small to be of statistical significance.

Results of the two treatments in cases with "malignant involvement" of Ohngren's criteria were also compared. In the treatment of cases with "malignant involvement" the 5-year survival rates of the AI series and no-AI series were 52% of 23 cases and 26% of 35 cases, respectively. This difference was also too small to be of statistical significance. However, this comparison suggested the superiority of arterial infusion combined treatment.

An advantage of arterial chemotherapy was also demonstrated in avoiding aggressive surgery. In the patients who had a T_{3b} or T_4 lesion and survived 5 years or more, 9 of 13 patients did not need total maxillectomy in the AI series, whereas only one out of 7 cases did not need total maxillectomy in the no-AI series.

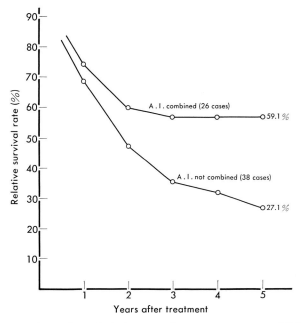

FIG. 2. Comparison of survivals between the two treatment modalities—combined and not combined with arterial infusion in the treatment of advanced cases (T_{3b}, T_4)

Late Effects and Complications

There is a risk of late radiation effects developing in the treated area. The incidence of these has been more frequent in this series than observed in other studies.

About 80% of the cases which were controlled for more than 3 years without extirpation of the orbit developed damage of the eye within 3 years after treatment. From our experience, the maximum dose of radiation which did not produce heavy damage of the eye was approximately 4,000 rad. This dose of radiation is not sufficient to eradicate squamous cell carcinoma completely.

Infection in the area irradiated may induce late radiation necrosis in the bone. This necrosis of the bone has often persisted for several years and was sometimes fatal. Seven patients died from intracranial infection following bone necrosis of the base of the skull without any evidence of persistent tumor on autopsy. All of these patients had advanced carcinoma involving a suprastructure or posterior structure and were treated by heavy external irradiation followed by total maxillectomy with extirpation of the orbit, and further, given intracavitary irradiation to prevent recurrence.

From these experiences, our main aim in the treatment of carcinoma of the maxillary sinus has been to keep the dose of radiation to less than 4,000 rad.

COMMENTS

In Europe and U.S.A., arterial chemotherapy combined with radiotherapy or surgery has not been generally accepted as the usual method for treatment of carcinoma of the maxillary sinus. In these countries, arterial infusion therapy has usually been used as palliation for advanced cases (*2, 4, 10*), and radiation therapy followed by aggressive surgery has been used as the most reliable method of treatment (*11*). In our country, however, arterial chemotherapy has generally been used as a routine method of treatment during recent years. Investigation of the patients in the National Cancer Center Hospital, Tokyo revealed some advantages of arterial chemotherapy combined with radiotherapy and surgery.

The most distinct advantage was observed in improvement of survival without aggressive surgery even in the treatment of advanced cases. As mentioned above, during the last 3 years we have made an effort to decrease the radiation dose to less than 4,000 rad by combining with arterial chemotherapy. From our experience, although the end-results have not yet been obtained, we have confidence that complications such as heavy damage to the orbit, production of necrosis in the bone for a prolonged period, and intracranial complications could be avoided without sacrificing the survival rate. The most dramatic advantage of this recent treatment could be found in rehabilitation of the patients. Duration of admission of the patients was distinctly decreased and the patients were able to live in almost the same condition as before suffering the disease.

REFERENCES

1. Frazell, E. L. and Levis, J. S. Cancer of the nasal cavity and accessory sinuses: A report of the management of 416 patients. *Cancer*, **16**, 1293 (1963).
2. Goepfert, H., Jesse, R. H., and Lindberg, R. D. Arterial infusion and radiation therapy

in the treatment of advanced cancer of the nasal cavity and paranasal sinuses. *Am. J. Surg.*, **126**, 474 (1973).

3. Jesse, R. H. Preoperative *versus* postoperative radiation in the treatment of squamous carcinoma of the paranasal sinuses. *Am. J. Surg.*, **110**, 552 (1965).

4. Jesse, R. H., Goepfert, H., and Lindberg, R. Squamous cell carcinoma of maxillary and ethmoid sinuses. *Proc. Natl Cancer Conf. 7th* (1973).

5. Larsson, L. G. and Martensson, G. Carcinoma of the paranasal sinus and the nasal cavities. *Acta Radiol.*, **42**, 149 (1954).

6. Macbeth, R. Malignant disease of the paranasal sinuses. *J. Laryngol.*, **79**, 592 (1965).

7. Marchetta, F. C., Sako, K., Mattick, W. L., and Stinziano, G. D. Squamous cell carcinoma of the maxillary antrum. *Am. J. Surg.*, **118**, 805 (1969).

8. Sakai, S., Fuchihata, H., and Hamasaki, Y. Treatment policy for maxillary sinus carcinoma. *Acta Otolaryngol.*, **82**, 172 (1976).

9. Sato, Y., Morita, M., Takahashi, H., Watanabe, N., and Kirikae, I. Combined surgery, radiotherapy and regional chemotherapy in carcinoma of the paranasal sinuses. *Cancer*, **25**, 571 (1970).

10. Sealy, R., Helman, P., Greenstein, A., and Shepstone B. The treatment of locally advanced cancer of the head and neck with intra-arterial cytotoxics, cobalt and hyperbaric oxygen therapy. *Cancer*, **34**, 497 (1974).

11. Tabb, H. G. and Branco, S. J. Cancer of the maxillary sinus: An analysis of 108 cases. *Laryngoscope*, **81**, 818 (1971).

CANCERS OF THE LARYNX AND HYPOPHARYNX

Ikuichiro Hɪʀoᴛo*¹ and Akinori Iᴄʜɪᴋᴀᴡᴀ*²

*Department of Otorhinolaryngology, Faculty of Medicine,
Kyushu University,*¹ and
Department of Otorhinolaryngology, School of Medicine,
Kurume University*²*

Five-year survival rate of 135 cases of laryngeal carcinoma which were treated during the 10 years from 1960–1969 was 70.4%. The result for supraglottic carcinoma was 59.5% and that of glottic carcinoma was 81.4%. Five-year survival rate in 35 cases that had radiation therapy, 30 cases having partial laryngectomy, and 75 cases having total laryngectomy were respectively 81.6%, 67.1%, and 64.2%.

Five-year survival rate of 33 cases of hypopharyngeal carcinoma was 33.9%.

One hundred and thirty-five cases of laryngeal carcinoma and 33 cases of laryngopharyngeal carcinoma were treated in the Kurume University Hospital during 10 years from January, 1960, to December, 1969. During this decade, the policy for selecting a therapeutic procedure in Japan has changed from extensive radical surgery for any case to conservative function-retaining surgery or radiation for selected cases. External fractionated radiotherapy used to be offered for early growths, especially for glottic carcinoma in Stage T_1, and it tended to be applied to more advanced growths in combination with chemotherapy. Partial laryngectomy came to be a routine technique for laryngeal carcinoma in its early stage in the latter half of this decade, and also larynx-preserving surgery was employed for hypopharyngeal carcinoma in its early stage instead of pharyngo-laryngoesophagectomy that had been the usual ordinary technique for any case of this carcinoma.

Methods of Studies

One hundred and thirty-five cases of laryngeal carcinoma consisted of 123 male cases (91%) and 12 females. The mean age of the 135 cases was 63 years, with a range of 38 to 80 years. Staging of these cases was made retrospectively according to the UICC classification of 1968. They were grouped into 59 cases of supraglottic carcinoma (43.7%), 68 cases of glottic carcinoma (50.4%), and 8 cases of subglottic carcinoma (5.9%). Primary tumors were classified into 32 cases of Stage T_1 (23.7%), 32 cases of Stage T_2, 57 cases of Stage T_3 (42.2%), and 14 cases of Stage T_4 (10.4%). The enlargement of cervical lymph nodes was noticed in 51 of 135 cases (37.8%).

The policy of treatment in this series was in principle as follows, being modified according to the patient's age, general health, and the patient's preference.

*¹ Maidashi 3-1-1, Higashi-ku, Fukuoka 812, Japan (広戸幾一郎).
*² Asahimachi 67, Kurume 830, Japan (市川昭則).

Irradiation was the first choice when the primary tumor was not so invasive and limited to one or two sites (glottic T_1, T_2, supraglottic T_1) without metastatic lymph nodes. Partial laryngectomy was performed when 1) the primary tumor was located at one or two sites in the supraglottic region and its extention was limited within the anterior one-third of both aryepiglottic folds, 2) the primary tumor was located in one side of the glottic region and showed few extensions to the other side, and an affected vocal cord might be impaired in its mobility but not fixed. 3) Metastatic lymph nodes might be found but movable in the diseased side. Total laryngectomy was primarily performed in advanced cases (T_2, T_3, T_4) and secondarily carried out when the tumor was not controlled by irradiation or partial laryngectomy. Radical neck dissection was always carried out when 1) metastatic lymph nodes were found, 2) total laryngectomy was performed for the recurrence of the primary tumor which was found after partial laryngectomy. Planned preoperative irradiation was not employed in these cases.

Thirty-three cases of hypopharyngeal carcinoma consisted of 18 male and 15 female cases. The mean age of the 33 cases was 58 years, with a range of 37 to 76 years. They were grouped into 11 cases of piriform sinus carcinoma, 14 cases of postcricoid carcinoma, and 8 cases of posterior wall carcinoma. The enlargement of regional lymph nodes was found in 17 of 33 cases (51.5%). Irradiation was made in 2 cases in compliance with the patient's preference. Pharyngo-esophagectomy was carried out in 9 selected early cases. Pharyngo-laryngo-esophagectomy was performed in 22 cases at any stage. Meanwhile, 9 cases (4 males and 5 females) of cervical esophagus carcinoma were treated in our clinic during the same decade.

Five-year survival rate for each group of laryngeal carcinoma was computed by the acturial, or life table, method. Computations were performed by recording for each 1-year interval of follow-up: 1) The number alive at the beginning of the interval, 2) the number that died during the interval, and 3) the number withdrawn alive or lost to follow-up during the interval. The observed 5-year cumulative survival rate was given by such computating procedures. The corrected or relative survival rate is defined as the ratio of the observed survival rate to the expected survival rate estimated through the use of a general population life table in Japan. Five-year survival rate in this study means the relative 5-year survival rate calculated by the acturial method.

Results

Out of 135 cases of laryngeal carcinoma, 31 cases (23%) died of local recurrence, cervical or lung metastasis, and 26 cases (19%) died of other causes within 5 years after treatment. The 5-year survival rate for this carcinoma is 70.4%. Out of 33 cases of hypopharyngeal carcinoma, 18 cases (55%) died of recurrent or metastatic carcinoma and 5 cases (15%) died of other causes during 5 years after treatment. The 5-year survival rate for this carcinoma is 33.9% (Table I).

The enlargement of cervical lymph nodes in laryngeal carcinoma was observed in 51 of 135 cases (37.8%). Five-year survival rate was 73.3% in these cases, and was 74.1% in 84 cases without lymph node enlargement. In hypopharyngeal carcinoma, palpable lymph nodes in the neck were found in 17 cases and not noted in 16 cases. Five-year survival rate was 36.0% in the former and 38.3% in the latter (Table II).

TABLE I. Five-year Survival Rate of Laryngeal and Hypopharyngeal Carcinomas

	Laryngeal	Hypopharyngeal
Number alive at the beginning	135	33
Number who died during the 5 years	57	23
Number lost to follow up during the 5 years	6	0
5-year survival rates (%)		
Observed	57.4	30.3
Expected	81.5	89.4
Relative	70.4	33.9
Standard deviation	80.8–60.0	51.7–16.1

TABLE II. Five-year Survival Rate related to Regional Lymph Nodes

	Laryngeal		Hypopharyngeal	
	N0	N+	N0	N+
Number of cases	84	51	16	17
5-Year relative survival rate (%)	74.1	73.3	38.3	36.0
Standard deviation	87.1–61.1	90.3–56.3	66.7–9.9	63.0–9.0

1. Supraglottic carcinoma

Fifty-nine cases (54 males and 5 females) with a supraglottic lesion were treated. The mean age of the 59 cases was 62 years, with a range of 38 to 79 years. Six were in Stage T_1, 22 in Stage T_2, 19 in Stage T_3, and 12 were Stage T_4.

Irradiation was the initial treatment in 6 early cases (3 each of Stage T_1, Stage T_2). Of them, one uncontrolled case underwent total laryngectomy but died of lung metastasis, one died of another cause, and one was lost to follow-up. Three of 6 cases (all Stage T_1) stayed alive for more than 5 years. Cure rate of the primary tumor was 5 out of 6, 83.3%.

Supraglottic horizontal laryngectomy was performed in 8 early cases (2 of Stage T_1 and 6 of Stage T_2) and subtotal laryngectomy with or without partial pharyngectomy was carried out in 2 advanced cases (T_3 and T_4). Of the former 8 cases, 3 cases died of other causes, 1 died of lung metastasis, and 2 underwent total laryngectomy but died of recurrence in the neck. The latter 2 cases were subsequently controlled by total laryngectomy and stayed alive for more than 5 years. Cure rate of the primary tumor was 6 out of 10, 60.0%.

Total laryngectomy was performed primarily in 43 cases (one of Stage T_1, 13 of Stage T_2, 18 of Stage T_3, and 11 of Stage T_4) and secondarily in 5 cases. Out of the primary 43 cases, 4 died of metastasis to the cervical lymph nodes, 6 died of lung metastasis, 9 died of other causes, and 2 cases of Stage T_4 died of local recurrence of the primary tumor. None was lost to follow-up. Twenty-two of 43 primary cases and 2 of 5 secondary cases stayed alive for more than 5 years after surgery. Five-year survival rate was 59.5% (75.3–43.7%) in 59 cases of supraglottic carcinoma.

2. Glottic carcinoma

Sixty-eight cases (62 males and 6 females) with glottic tumor were treated. The mean age of the 68 cases was 63 years, with a range of 39 to 80 years. Twenty-six were in Stage T_1, 10 in Stage T_2, 31 in Stage T_3, and one in Stage T_4.

Irradiation was initially made in 29 cases. Twenty-one were observed after irradiation without surgery. They were composed of 15 cases of Stage T_1, 4 of Stage T_2, and 2 of Stage T_3. Of these, one died of local recurrence of the primary tumor, one died of lung metastasis, 5 died from other causes, and 2 were lost to follow-up. Fifteen of 21 cases remained alive without disease. The other 8 of 29 cases were not controlled by irradiation and were retreated surgically. They were 5 cases of Stage T_1, 2 cases of Stage T_2, and 1 case of Stage T_3. Frontolateral laryngectomy was performed in 4 cases and total laryngectomy in the other 4 cases. Of these, 2 cases died of lung metastasis, one died from another cause, and one was lost to follow-up. Half stayed alive for more than 5 years. The cure rate of the primary tumor was 20 out of 29, 68.9%.

Frontolateral laryngectomy was done primarily in 14 cases (5 of Stage T_1, one of Stage T_2, and 8 of Stage T_3) and secondarily in 4 cases which were not controlled by irradiation (3 of Stage T_1, one of Stage T_2). Of the former 14 cases, one died from another cause and 4 were submitted to total laryngectomy due to recurrence of the primary tumor; on the other hand, one case died from another cause and one was lost to follow up in the latter 4 cases. The cure rate of the primary tumor was 10 out of 14, 71.4% in the primarily laryngectomized cases and 14 out of 18, 77.8% in all cases including the secondarily laryngectomized cases.

Total laryngectomy was carried out initially in 25 cases (one of Stage T_1, 3 of Stage T_2, 20 of Stage T_3, and one of Stage T_4) and secondarily in 8 cases. Of the initial 25 cases, one died of local recurrence of the primary tumor, 3 died of metastasis to the cervical lymph nodes, 5 died from other causes, and 2 were lost to follow-up. All those who died belonged to the Stage T_3 group. In the secondary 8 cases, 3 died of recurrence in the metastatic cervical lymph node and one died from another cause. Fourteen of 25 primary cases and 4 of 8 secondary cases lived without disease for more than 5 years. Five-year survival rate was 81.4% (95.6–67.2%) in 68 cases of glottic carcinoma.

3. Subglottic carcinoma

Eight cases (7 males and 1 female) with subglottic growth were treated. The mean age of the 8 cases was 64 years, with a range of 47 to 77 years. Seven were Stage T_3 and one was Stage T_4.

Irradiation was not employed in these cases. Vertical hemilaryngectomy was performed in one case of Stage T_3, who died from local recurrence of the primary tumor. Total laryngectomy was carried out in 7 cases (6 of Stage T_3, one of Stage T_4), 2 cases of which died of recurrence in metastatic cervical lymph nodes and one died of lung metastasis. Five-year survival rate was 70.4% (103.7–17.7%) in 8 cases of subglottic carcinoma.

4. Total outcome

Observed 5-year survival rate in the T-classification was 94.2% in the Stage T_1 group, 58.0% in the Stage T_2 group, 73.8% in the Stage T_3 group, and 41.0% in the Stage T_4 group, as shown in Table III. The survival rate of the Stage T_2 group was worse than that of the Stage T_3 group. It is difficult to elucidate this reason clearly, but the T-classification table of 1968 may not be entirely adequate.

TABLE III. Five-year Survival Rate of Laryngeal Carcinoma Related
to Its Region and Extension

Stage	T_1	T_2	T_3	T_4	Total (%)
Supraglottic	5/6	7/22	12/19	4/12	28/59 (59.5)
Glottic	17/26	6/10	16/31	1/1	40/68 (81.4)
Subglottic	—	—	4/7	0/1	4/8 (70.4)
Total (%)	22/32 (94.2)	13/32 (58.0)	32/57 (73.8)	5/14 (41.0)	72/135 (70.4)

Radiation therapy was initially employed in 35 cases, of which 9 cases were surgically retreated due to the failure of irradiation and 26 cases were observed without surgery. Five-year survival rate of the 35 irradiated cases was 81.6% (101.9–61.2%), which was 86.3% (109.9–62.7%) in 26 cases treated by irradiation alone.

Partial laryngectomy was initially performed in 25 cases and secondarily in 5 cases which were not controlled by irradiation. Of these 30 cases, 9 cases were submitted to total laryngectomy due to recurrence of the primary tumor. Five-year survival rate of the 30 partially laryngectomized cases was 67.1% (88.8–45.3%), 75.4% (102.4–48.4%) in 17 cases treated only by partial laryngectomy.

Total laryngectomy was primarily done in 75 cases and secondarily in 13 cases which were not controlled by irradiation or partial laryngectomy. Five-year survival rate was 64.2% (77.0–51.3%) in all 88 cases, 67.4% in the primary 75 cases, and 46.0% in the 13 cases secondarily laryngectomized.

Elective neck dissection was performed in 35 of 84 cases in which cervical lymph node was not palpable but the primary tumor of the larynx looked invasive. In supraglottic carcinoma, cervical recurrence was observed in one of 13 cases which underwent elective neck dissection (7.6%), and cervical metastasis became manifest later in 4 of 16 cases which were observed without elective neck dissection (25.0%). In glottic and subglottic carcinomas, recurrence after neck dissection was found in 6 of 22 cases (27.2%), and cervical metastasis was revealed in 5 of 33 cases without elective neck dissection (15.1%). It was notable that 1) 5 of 9 recurrent cases died of lung metastasis when elective neck dissection was not performed, 2) recurrence in paratracheal lymph nodes was observed in 4 of 6 recurrent cases of glottic and subglottic carcinomas when elective neck dissection was performed.

Therapeutic neck dissection is a routine procedure for the enlargement of cervical lymph nodes, but was not carried out when palpable lymph nodes were considered not to be metastatic. In supraglottic carcinoma, cervical recurrence was observed in 4 of 22 cases which were submitted to therapeutic neck dissection (18.1%), and cervical metastasis became manifest later in 3 of 8 cases in which neck dissection was not performed (37.0%). In glottic and subglottic carcinomas, recurrence in the neck was found in 3 of 18 cases with neck dissection (16.6%) and in 2 of 3 cases without neck dissection (66.6%). It was noted that 1) recurrence after neck dissection was chiefly found in the upper jugular lymph nodes in supraglottic carcinoma and in the paratracheal lymph nodes in glottic and subglottic carcinomas, 2) lung metastasis was observed only in cases without therapeutic neck dissection.

TABLE IV. Recurrence or Metastasis of the Tumor Related to Neck Dissection

Cervical lymph node	Region of the tumor	Neck dissection	No. of recurrence	Site of recurrence or metastasis	Prognosis
N0	Supraglottic	Done	1/13	Upper jugular	Alive
		Not done	4/16	Upper jugular	Dead
				3 Lung metastasis	All dead
	Glottic and subglottic	Done	6/22	2 Upper jugular	One dead
				4 Paratracheal	2 dead
		Not done	5/33	3 Upper jugular	One dead
				2 Lung metastasis	2 dead
N+	Supraglottic	Done	4/22	4 Upper jugular	All dead
		Not done	3/8	3 Upper jugular	2 dead
	Glottic and subglottic	Done	3/18	3 Paratracheal	All dead
		Not done	2/3	Upper jugular	Alive
				Lung metastasis	Alive

5. Hypopharyngeal carcinoma

The mean age of the 11 cases (10 males and 1 female) with piriform sinus lesion was 63 years, with a range of 48 to 76 years; that of the 14 cases (4 males and 10 females) with postcricoid lesion was 57 years, with a range of 37 to 65 years; that of the 8 cases (4 males and 4 females) with posterior wall lesion was 54 years, with a range of 49 to 62 years. Four were Stage T_1, 7 in Stage T_2, and 22 in Stage T_3.

Irradiation was carried out in 2 cases (Stage T_2 and T_3 of piriform sinus carcinoma), both of which died of local recurrence of the primary tumor and some other cause. Pharyngo-esophagectomy, preserving the larynx, was carried out in 9 cases (one of Stage T_2 of piriform sinus carcinoma, one of Stage T_1 of postcricoid carcinoma, 2 of Stage T_1, 1 of Stage T_2, and 4 of Stage T_3 of posterior wall carcinoma). Of these, 4 cases died of local recurrence of the primary tumor, one died of recurrence in the cervical lymph node, and one died from another cause. Pharyngolaryngo-esophagectomy was performed in 22 cases (one of Stage T_1, 1 of Stage T_2, and 6 of Stage T_3 of piriform sinus carcinoma, 3 of Stage T_2 and 10 of Stage T_3 of postcricoid carcinoma, and 1 of Stage T_3 of posterior wall carcinoma). Of these, 5 cases died of local recurrence of the primary tumor, 4 died of recurrence in the cervical lymph node, 3 died of lung metastasis, and 3 died from other causes.

Five-year survival rate in pharyngo-esophagectomy was 37.2% and that of pharyngo-laryngo-esophagectomy was 35.2%. The result of piriform sinus carcinoma was the best and that of postcricoid carcinoma was the worst; that is, the 5-year survival rate was 44.4% in the former, 23.1% in the latter, and 39.9% in posterior wall carcinoma. Meanwhile, the 5-year survival rate was 36.8% in 9 cases of cervical esophagus carcinoma.

DISCUSSION

The frequency rate of supraglottic carcinoma to glottic carcinoma is usually 35 to 65% in western countries as presented by MacComb and others (7). This ratio is

46 to 54% in our experience and 49 to 51% in Fujimaki's nationwide statistics of 6,360 cases in Japan (1). It is a peculiarity of laryngeal carcinoma in Japan that supraglottic carcinoma is in the majority.

The prognosis of laryngeal cancer is fairly satisfactory compared with that of other cancers. Five-year survival rate was 70.4% in our 135 cases and 62.1% in 6,360 cases treated during the same decade in Japan. The result is generally better in glottic carcinoma than in supraglottic one. Five-year survival rate was 81.4% in glottic carcinoma and 59.5% in supraglottic carcinoma in our cases; it was 76.1% in the former and 50.7% in the latter in Fujimaki's nationwide statistics of Japan (1).

It has been difficult to compare the results of radiation therapy and surgery for laryngeal carcinoma because they have been separately presented by radiologists and surgeons. Irradiation and partial laryngectomy have both been indicated for early cases of laryngeal carcinoma such as Stage T_1 and T_2. A strictly determined indication of partial laryngectomy has been similar to that of irradiation. Our experience led us to the following policy on this subject.

In glottic carcinoma, irradiation should be the treatment of choice for Stage T_1 and T_2 lesions in which the vocal fold is movable, since the survival rate after irradiation was not so different from that of partial laryngectomy and the vocal quality was better in successfully irradiated cases than in those partially laryngectomized cases. Partial laryngectomy, such as vertical hemilaryngectomy, should preferentially be performed for some cases of Stage T_3 and T_2 lesions in which the mobility of the vocal fold is impaired.

In supraglottic carcinoma, irradiation should be preferred to partial laryngectomy for a Stage T_1 lesion due to its far better result than that of partial laryngectomy. For a Stage T_2 lesion, it is expected to be functionally most effective to perform supraglottic horizontal laryngectomy with planned preoperative irradiation.

Total laryngectomy was used for more advanced cases or recurrent cases after failure of irradiation or partial laryngectomy. Complete and careful neck dissection should always be performed with total laryngectomy for recurrent cases, that is, to remove paratracheal lymph nodes in glottic and subglottic carcinomas and upper jugular lymph nodes with a submandibular gland in supraglottic carcinoma whether palpable lymph nodes are found or not. In general, the result of secondary total laryngectomy which is performed after failure of irradiation is worse than that of initial total laryngectomy but better than that of total laryngectomy subsequently performed after failure of partial laryngectomy.

The rate of no recurrence or no metastasis was 82.5% in 40 cases which underwent therapeutic neck dissection and 54.5% in 11 cases without therapeutic neck dissection; however, there was no difference between 35 cases of elective neck dissection (80.0%) and 49 cases without elective neck dissection (81.6%). Reed (9) considered the immunological advantage of not removing regional lymph nodes until they are clinically involved and reassessed elective neck dissection since 70 out of 100 patients with carcinoma of the larynx may undergo unnecessary neck dissection to save, at the most, 8 patients.

In our policy, elective neck dissection is not always necessary for such cases as can be periodically examined after surgery. The rate of cervical metastasis found later in cases without elective neck dissection was less than 20% in our series. Such a metastasis in cervical lymph nodes can be sufficiently controlled by secondary therapeutic neck dissection if it is performed just after the detection of recurrence in the neck; however, it will be occasionally impossible to prevent lung metastasis when therapeutic neck dissection is delayed after recurrence. Therefore, elective neck dissection should always be performed at the initial surgery when the periodical examination is difficult. Although the periodical examination is possible, elective neck dissection should be done particularly for advanced cases above Stage T_3 in supraglottic carcinoma, because it showed a marked effect in preventing the recurrence in cervical lymph nodes. On the contrary, it showed little effect in glottic carcinoma. It is a good policy in this case to watch a patient without elective neck dissection.

CONCLUSIONS

1) Five-year survival rate of 135 cases of laryngeal carcinoma which were treated during the 10 years from 1960 to 1969 was 70.4% (standard deviation 80.8 to 60.0%). The results of radiation therapy in 35 cases, partial laryngectomy in 30 cases and total laryngectomy in 75 cases were respectively 81.6%, 67.1%, and 64.2%.

2) In glottic carcinoma, irradiation should be indicated to Stage T_1 and T_2 lesions and partial laryngectomy to Stage T_2 and T_3.

3) In supraglottic carcinoma, irradiation should be the treatment of choice for Stage T_1 lesion and partial laryngectomy for Stage T_2.

4) Elective neck dissection is not necessary in glottic carcinoma; however, it should be done for advanced cases above Stage T_3 in supraglottic carcinoma.

5) Five-year survival rate of 33 cases of hypopharyngeal carcinoma was 33.9% (standard deviation was 51.7% to 16.1%).

REFERENCES

1. Fujimaki, T. A clinical study on statistics of laryngeal cancer in Japan 1960–1969. *Nihon Jibiinkokagakkai Kaiho (Japan. J. Otol., Tokyo)*, **76**, 533–577 (1973) (in Japanese).
2. Hiroto, I. Hypopharyngoesophageal carcinoma, its surgical treatment. *Kurume Med. J.*, **10**, 162–172 (1963).
3. Hiroto, I. Partial laryngectomy. *Jibi Inkoka Rinsho (Pract. Otol., Kyoto)*, **58**, 178–189 (1965) (in Japanese).
4. Hiroto, I. Pathological studies relating to neoplasms of the hypopharynx and the cervical esophagus. *Kurume Med. J.*, **16**, 127–133, 1969.
5. Leonard, J. R. and Litton, W. B. Selection of the patient for conservation surgery of the larynx. *Laryngoscope*, **81**, 232–252 (1971).
6. Leronx-Robert, J. Indications et résultats aprés 5 ans de la chirurgie conservatrice fonctionnelle des cancers du larynx et de l'hypopharynx. *Adv. Oto-Rhino-Laryngol.*, **9**, 44–130 (1961).
7. MacComb, W. S. "Cancer of the Head and Neck," The Williams and Wilkins Co., Baltimore (1967).
8. Ogura, J. H. Supraglottic subtotal laryngectomy and radical neck dissection for carcinoma of the epiglottis. *Laryngoscope*, **68**, 983–1003 (1958).
9. Reed, F. G. and Miller, W. A. Elective neck dissection. *Laryngoscope*, **80**, 1292–1304 (1970).

CANCER OF THE THYROID

Rikio FURIHATA, Masao MAKIUCHI, Makoto MIYAKAWA,
and Nobuyuki KAWAMURA

*Department of Surgery, Faculty of Medicine, Shinshu University**

A retrospective analysis of surgical treatment, recurrent disease, and carcinoma death in thyroid carcinoma, which was treated at the Shinshu University Hospital for 23 years, has been reported. The results of follow-up study of 592 patients with thyroid carcinoma revealed that there were some obvious differences between adenocarcinoma and anaplastic carcinoma in biologic behavior, response to treatment, and prognosis. The following policy of surgical treatment for thyroid carcinoma is recomended.

1. The most adequate procedure for adenocarcinoma is surgical excision.

   1) For removal of primary tumor of the thyroid, lobectomy or more extensive resection is preferable.

   2) Modified radical neck dissection, including the jugular vein but preserving the sternocleidomastoid muscle, is the treatment of choice for regional lymph node metastasis.

2. Combination therapy with surgical excision and irradiation may be indicated for anaplastic carcinoma at the present time, though its prognosis is very poor.

Surgical excision is generally recognized as the primary treatment for thyroid carcinoma. However, there has been some controversy over the amount of thyroid tissue which should be excised and the management of the cervical lymph nodes: Some surgeons (2, 4) have favored conservative procedures, but others (3, 5) have advocated radical surgery.

This paper presents cases of thyroid carcinoma seen for their pathological diagnosis and surgical treatment at the Shinshu University Hospital from 1953 to 1975. In an attempt to evaluate the effect of surgical treatment on the course of the carcinoma, the pathogenesis of recurrence and carcinoma death have been related to the extent of the primary surgery.

Clinical Cases

Five hundred and ninety-two cases of thyroid carcinoma were primarily diagnosed and treated at the Shinshu University Hospital in the 23 years during 1953–1975. The pathological classification of the carcinomas by Meissner and Warren (7) is listed in Table I. Papillary adenocarcinoma and follicular adenocarcinoma were mostly seen in

---

* Asahi 3-1-1, Matsumoto, Nagano 390, Japan (降旗力男, 牧内正夫, 宮川 信, 川村信之).

TABLE I. Pathological Classification of Thyroid Carcinoma

Histological type	No. of patients
Papillary adenocarcinoma	522
Follicular adenocarcinoma	44
Anaplastic carcinoma	21
Squamous cell carcinoma	4
Medullary carcinoma	1
Total	592

the age groups of 30 to 50 years, but anaplastic carcinoma and squamous cell carcinoma were seen in the age groups over 50 years.

Surgical treatment was performed as a radical procedure in 520 and as a palliative procedure in 72 of 592 cases. Survival rates were calculated by the method of relative survival rate (1, 6).

Follow-up Data

Five hundred and thirty-eight of 592 cases were traced after surgery for the entire period, but 54 cases (53 papillary and 1 follicular adenocarcinoma) were lost. The results of surgical treatment for adenocarcinoma and anaplastic carcinoma are summarized in Table II. Generally, survival rates of papillary adenocarcinoma are fairly good and those of anaplastic carcinoma are very poor. It is noteworthy that 10- and 15-year survival rates of papillary adenocarcinoma after palliative operation are 74.9% and 53.0%, respectively. It was also observed in adenocarcinoma that comparing the 2 groups of younger patients (under 50 years of age) and older patients (more than 50 years of age), 10- and 15-year survival rates of the younger group are 100.7% and 100.0%, respectively, but those of the older group are 95.9% and 81.2%, respectively (Table III). Namely, the prognosis of younger patients with adenocarcinoma of the thyroid is better than that of older patients.

TABLE II. Survival Rates after Surgical Treatment Calculated
by Relative Survival Rate (1, 6)

Survival period (years)	Radical operation (%)			Palliative operation (%)		
	Papillary adenocarcinoma	Follicular adenocarcinoma	Anaplastic carcinoma	Papillary adenocarcinoma	Follicular adenocarcinoma	Anaplastic carcinoma
5	99.9	90.0	0	73.7	34.7	0
10	97.4	82.1	0	74.9	0	0
15	99.3	82.1	0	53.0	0	0

TABLE III. Comparison of Survival Rates between Younger and Older Patients
with Papillary Adenocarcinoma after Radical Surgery

Survival period (years)	50 years and under (321 patients) (%)	Over 50 years (187 patients) (%)
10	100.7	95.9
15	100.0	81.2

These results suggest that there are some obvious differences in biological behavior and therefore in the response to treatment and prognosis between adenocarcinoma and anaplastic carcinoma of the thyroid.

Cause of Death

It was sometimes difficult to determine a single cause of death. As is true of many morbid conditions, secondary complications or subsequent disease often contributed to death in this series of patients. Immediate cause of death among the patients who clearly died of thyroid carcinoma is summarized in Table IV.

Eight patients with papillary adenocarcinoma died primarily of respiratory obstruction due to locally recurrent tumor and 8 patients died of inanition with lung and/or bone metastasis. Five patients with follicular adenocarcinoma died of distant metastases and 1 patient died of massive bleeding from a recurrent tumor in the neck. Six patients with anaplastic carcinoma died of distant metastases and 4 patients clearly died of respiratory obstruction or bleeding due to a recurrent tumor in the neck.

As respiratory obstruction or massive bleeding due to a recurrent tumor is regarded as one of the most common causes of death in thyroid carcinoma, consideration must be given to the surgical procedure to minimize postoperative recurrence in the neck, especially around the cervical trachea.

TABLE IV. Cause of Death after Radical Surgery for Thyroid Carcinoma

Cause of death	No. of patients		
	Papillary adenocarcinoma	Follicular adenocarcinoma	Anaplastic carcinoma
Respiratory obstruction	8	0	3
Distant metastasis	8	5	6
Massive bleeding	0	1	1
Others	7	1	3
Total	23	7	13

Surgical Procedures

Owing to lower radiosensitivity and lower efficacy of anticancer drugs, surgical excision is the treatment of choice for adenocarcinoma. On the other hand, combination therapy with surgical excision and irradiation may be the optimum choice for anaplastic carcinoma, which has a higher radiosensitivity.

Surgical procedures used for adenocarcinoma at the Shinshu University Hospital are discussed as follows.

1. Tumor removal

Several procedures are used to remove thyroid tumors, and their selection depends on the size of tumor and the extent of its invasion to the surrounding tissues. Lobectomy is performed most frequently, with additional isthmectomy carried out when necessary. Indication for subtotal thyroidectomy or partial lobectomy is very limited, and total thyroidectomy was performed in 13 advanced cases. Enucleation was performed to

TABLE V. Surgical Procedures for Adenocarcinoma and Postoperative Recurrence

Procedure	No. of patients	Incidence of recurrence (%)
Total thyroidectomy	13	0
Subtotal thyroidectomy	23	4.3
Lobectomy	289	2.8
Partial lobectomy	28	3.6
Enucleation	76	9.2

remove the very small and well-localized tumor in the unilateral lobe initially in this series (Table V).

There were no recurrences in the remnant after total thyroidectomy, but some were revealed in 8 of 289 cases (2.8%) after lobectomy, with or without isthmectomy, in 1 of 28 cases (3.6%) after partial lobectomy, and in 1 of 23 cases (4.3%) after subtotal thyroidectomy. Lobectomy or more extensive resection of the thyroid is thus an essential clinical procedure.

2. Surgical procedure for adhesion or invasion of thyroid tumor to the surrounding tissues

Adhesion of the tumor to the surrounding tissues existed in 74.4% of adenocarcinomas. Higher incidences of adhesion were seen with the anterior cervical muscles (58.5%), with the trachea (47.5%), and with the esophagus (16.3%). From the standpoint of postoperative recurrence, the treatment for tracheal adhesion or invasion is most important. Actually, separation of a slightly adherent tumor from the trachea was performed in 212 cases with relative ease, and 186 patients still survive. However, 11 patients died of thyroid carcinoma, and another 6 are alive with local recurrence of carcinoma (Table VI).

Residual carcinoma tissue, on the tracheal wall, was cauterized in 18 cases after removal of the primary tumor: 13 of 18 patients are doing well and 3 others survived

TABLE VI. Surgical Procedure for Adhesion or Invasion
of Thyroid Tumor to the Tracheal Wall

Procedure	No. of patients	No. of patients alive	
		Doing well	With recurrence
Removal of tumor from the trachea alone	212	186	6
Cauterization on the tracheal wall	18	13	3
Curettage on the tracheal wall	4	0	3
Partial resection of the tracheal wall	1	1	0
Combined resection of the larynx and trachea	1	1	0

TABLE VII. Procedures of Regional Lymph Node Dissection and Recurrence

Procedure	No. of patients	Incidence of recurrence (%)
Modified radical neck dissection	170	9.4
Excision of enlarged nodes alone	65	15.4
Resection of primary tumor alone	194	5.2

with local recurrences. Curettage of the residual carcinoma tissue on the tracheal wall was performed in 4 patients, but the results were poor; one died and the other 3 had local recurrences (Table VI).

Partial resection of the trachea or extensive resection including the larynx was attempted in cases with invasion of cancer onto the inner surface of the trachea. However, the operative indication of these aggressive procedures is very rare in adenocarcinomas of the thyroid (Table VI).

3. Lymph node dissection

Modified radical neck dissection was performed in 170 cases with multiple cervical lymph node metastases. Excision of the involving nodes alone was performed in 65 cases. In 194 cases without any cervical node involvement preoperatively, resection of the primary tumor alone was performed (Table VII).

Recurrence of lymph node metastasis was seen in 9.4% of patients after modified radical neck dissection. Higher incidence of recurrence (15.4%) was found in patients treated only by local excision of involved lymph nodes. Recurrence of regional lymph node metastasis occurred in 5.2% of patients after resection of only the primary tumor (Table VII).

Modified radical neck dissection is apparently the first choice of treatment for lymph node metastasis. However, local dissection is not an adequate procedure for the patient with lymph node metastasis.

Complete histopathological examination of dissected cervical lymph node was made in 69 cases after modified radical neck dissection. The incidence of lymph node metastasis was 69.6% in the inferior deep cervical node, 63.7% in the paratracheal node, 55.1% in the superior deep cervical node, and 43.5% in the pretracheal node. These results emphasize more extensive use of *en bloc* dissection of regional lymph nodes including the internal jugular vein.

The relationship between the localization of the primary tumor and regional lymph node metastasis was also examined. In cases with tumor growing in the entire lobe or at the upper or middle portion of the thyroid, lymph node metastasis developed widely from the superior to the inferior deep cervical node. On the other hand, patients with tumor that developed in the lower portion of the thyroid were likely to have lymph node metastasis more frequently in the inferior deep cervical node than in the superior one.

CONCLUSIONS

1. The following surgical procedures are recommended for the treatment of adenocarcinoma of the thyroid:
1) For removal of primary tumor of the thyroid, lobectomy or more extensive resection is preferable. 2) Owing to higher incidence of respiratory obstruction due to marked enlargement of the recurrent tumor, complete removal of the primary tumor around the trachea is the most important primary treatment. If the carcinoma has or is suspected to have invaded the surface of the tracheal wall, cauterization of residual cancer tissue is an effective procedure. 3) Modified radical neck dissection is the treatment of choice for regional lymph node metastasis. From the standpoint of surgical practice

more attention should be paid to prevent residual lymph node metastasis especially in the superior deep cervical node.

2. Combination therapy with surgical excision and irradiation for anaplastic carcinoma is indicated at the present time, though its prognosis is very poor.

REFERENCES

1. Berkson, J. and Gage, R. P. Calculation of survival rates for cancer. *Proc. Staff Meet. Mayo Clin.*, **25**, 270–286 (1950).
2. Buckwalter, J. A. and Thomas, C. G. Selection of surgical treatment for well-differentiated thyroid carcinomas. *Ann. Surg.*, **176**, 565–578 (1972).
3. Calcock, B. P. and Cattel, R. B. Carcinoma of the thyroid. *Surg. Clin. North Am.*, **42**, 687–691 (1962).
4. Crile, G., Jr. Late results of treatment for papillary cancer of the thyroid. *Ann. Surg.*, **160**, 178–182 (1964).
5. James, A. G. The management of papillary carcinoma of the thyroid gland. *Surgery*, **43**, 423–427 (1958).
6. Kurihara, M. and Takano, A. Computing method of the relative survival rate. *Gan-no-Rinsho (Cancer Clinic)*, **11**, 628–632 (1965) (in Japanese).
7. Meissner, W. A. and Warren, S. "Tumor of Thyroid Gland," Armed Forces Institute of Pathology, Washington, D.C. (1969).

CANCER OF THE THORACIC ESOPHAGUS

Komei NAKAYAMA

*Institute of Gastroenterology, Tokyo Women's Medical College**

The recent improvement in operative results is astonishing, and is largely due to extensive surgical experience, many good techniques, and development of anesthesia and antibiotics. However, from the aspect of completely curing cancer, the survival results should be considered, because some patients die after metastasis and relapse of cancer. The end results of esophageal cancer have not so far been satisfactory yet.

We have reviewed, and report here the 5-year survival results of resection of esophageal cancer in the Second Surgical Dept., Chiba University, and those in Tokyo Women's Medical College.

Generally speaking, esophageal cancer occurs more frequently in men, but the 5-year survival rate is a little better in women. The 5-year survival of males is 19.5% and of females is 23.5%. We have reviewed and reported the 5-year survival of cases after operation of thoracic esophageal carcinoma, as well as many other factors, sex, age, location of the lesion, length, type of X-ray examination, operative method, pathological findings, and so on.

Finally the number of patients alive for more than 10 years with upper or mid-thoracic esophageal cancer 40 and in lower esophageal cancer there were 83. After 20 years there were 4 upper and mid-thoracic esophageal cancer and 5 lower esophageal cancer patients still alive.

The findings of these cases indicate that esophageal cancer cannot be cured completely merely by improvement of the operative technique. The development of combined therapy with radiation or anticancer chemotherapy and immunotherapy will be required. Furthermore, the essential challenge to the disease "cancer" itself is required, and is the real problem in the future.

Seo (*11*) reviewed world literature on the resection of thoracic and abdominal esophageal cancer and reported in 1932 that of 151 cases, surgical death occurred in 144 and the mortality rate was 95.4%. According to the operative results of thoracic esophageal cancer in this Institute, in the period from February, 1965 to December, 1975, 29 of 671 cases died after surgery, and the mortality rate was 4.3%, which is an astonishing improvement. It is largely due to the accumulation of extensive surgical experience and the development of anesthesia and antibiotics. The end result should be considered in relation to the complete cure of cancer, because some patients may die due to metastasis or relapse of cancer. However, the end results of the treatment of esophageal cancer have not yet been satisfactory (*2, 10*). It is important to study the clinical aspects, to determine what patients can survive for a long time by

---

* Kawada-cho 10, Shinjuku-ku, Tokyo 162, Japan (中山恒明).

what type of treatment. We reviewed the 5-year survival results of surgery of eso-phageal cancer in the Second Surgical Department, Chiba University, and those in Tokyo Women's Medical College, and report them here.

Radical Operation of Esophageal Cancer

The subjects were patients with esophageal cancer who came to the Second Sur-gical Department, Chiba University, during 1946–1964, and those who were subjected to resection of esophageal cancer in the Institute of Gastroenterology, Tokyo Women's Medical College from February, 1965, to the end of December, 1970. As a result of progress in surgical technique, the operative results of esophageal cancer have im-proved; for example, the operative mortality was 4.2% in antethoracic reconstruction and 5.1% in intrathoracic reconstruction in the period from February, 1965 to 1975 (Table I), while they were 6.7% and 10.5%, respectively, in the period from 1946 to 1964 (6). Surgical death has decreased to nearly one-half during the past 10 years. When discussing the end result which can be obtained after long-term observation, as for 5 years, it is not possible to stop surgeons changing their concept of the opera-tion technique or therapy. Accordingly, though the subjects totalled 1,252 cases during the period of 1946–1975, the end results of 239 cases during 1965–1970 will be dis-cussed chiefly as newer data (2), the results of other cases will be shown where they are considered necessary.

TABLE I. Operative Results for Carcinoma of Upper and Mid-thoracic Esophagus

	No. of cases	Operative deaths	Mortality (%)
1946–1964			
Ante-thoracic reconstructed	503	34	6.7
Intra-thoracic reconstructed	75	8	10.5
Pull-through method	3	1	33.3
Total	581	43	7.4
1965–1975			
Ante-thoracic reconstructed	481	20	4.2
Intra-thoracic reconstructed	175	9	5.1
Retro-sternal reconstructed	15	0	0
Total	671	29	4.3

Sex, Age, and End Result

Sex and end result: Esophageal cancer occurs more frequently in males but the 5-year survival was a little better in females (Table II).

TABLE II. Sex and 5-Year Survivals (1965–1970)

	No. of cases	No. of 5-year survivals	Crude survival rate (%)
Males	205	40	19.5
Females	34	8	23.5
Total	239	48	20.0

TABLE III. Age and 5-Year Survivals (1965–1970)

Age (years)	No. of cases	No. of 5-year survivals	Crude survival rate (%)
–39	4	1	25.0
40–49	31	6	19.3
50–59	73	17	23.2
60–69	122	23	18.8
70–	9	1	11.1

Age and end result: No correlation was seen between age and 5-year survival (Table III).

X-Ray Findings and End Result

1. Location of lesion

In order to describe the location of lesion by X-ray examination, the thoracic esophagus was classified into the upper, middle, and lower parts according to the Descriptive Rules in Clinics and Pathology of Carcinoma of the Esophagus proposed by The Japanese Society of Esophageal Disease (*3*) as shown below. Although the 5-year survival is a little higher in Iu cases, correlation with the location of lesion was not as significant, considering that the number of subjects was small and included some early cancer cases (Table IV).

Upper thoracic esophagus (Iu)—From the upper side of the sternum to the lower side of the bifurcation of the trachea.

Middle thoracic esophagus (Im)—The upper half of the area from the lower end of the bifurcation of the trachea to the esophagocardiac junction.

Lower thoracic esophagus (Ei)—The intrathoracic esophagus in the lower half of the area from the lower end of the bifurcation of the trachea to the esophagocardiac junction.

TABLE IV. Location of the Lesion and 5-Year Survivals (1965–1970)

	No. of cases	No. of 5-year survivals	Crude survival rate (%)
Iu (upper thoracic esophagus)	7	3	42.8
Im (middle thoracic esophagus)	137	24	17.5
Ei (lower thoracic esophagus)	72	17	23.6
Ea (abdominal esophagus)	23	4	17.3

2. Length of filling defects

The relation of the length of filling defects to the 5-year survival rate was studied. The survival rate was similar untill the length reached 8 cm, but it decreased at greater lengths (Table V). According to the relationship between the length of filling defects and invasion to adventitia in the cases recently examined, many cases having defects shorter than 4 cm were a_0 and a_1, while those having defects longer than 8 cm were a_2 and a_3. In particular, there were 54% of a_3 cases, but no case having defects longer than

TABLE V. Length of Tumor (by X-ray Examination) and 5-Year Survivals (1965-1970)

Length of tumor (cm)	No. of cases	No. of 5-year survivals	Crude survival rate (%)
– 4.0	22	5	23
4.1– 6.0	87	20	23
6.1– 8.0	85	17	20
8.1–10.0	30	4	13
10.1–	14	2	14

TABLE VI. Relationship between the Length of Lesions by X-ray Examination and Grade of Invasion to Adventitia (1965-1975)

Length of lesion by X-ray (cm)	No. of cases	a_0 (%)	a_1 (%)	a_2 (%)	a_3 (%)
– 4.0	14	50	14	28	8
4.1– 6.0	77	19	9	48	24
6.1– 8.0	100	8	16	45	31
8.1–10.0	45	4	18	31	47
10.1	24	0	17	29	54

10 cm was a_0. The length of filling defects appeared to be proportional to the progress of cancer (Table VI).

3. Types of X-ray pictures

The Japanese Society of Esophageal Disease classifies the types of esophageal cancer observed on X-ray pictures into the following five: Superficial, tumorous, serrated, funnelled, and spiral. In relation to the type of disease, prognosis of the spiral type was the worst, while those of the superficial type and the tumorous type were better (4), because the latter two types were sharply demarcated and did not invade

TABLE VII. Type of the Lesions by X-ray Examination and 5-Year Survival Rate (1965-1970)

Type by X-ray	No. of cases	No. of 5-year survivals	Crude survival rate (%)
Superficial	7	5	71.4
Tumorous	7	3	42.8
Serrated	166	35	21.0
Funnelled	19	3	15.7
Spiral	35	2	5.7
Miscellaneous	5	0	0

TABLE VIII. Relation of the Type of Lesions by X-ray Examination and Grade of Invasion to Adventitia (1965-1975)

Type by X-ray	No. of cases	a_0 (%)	a_1 (%)	a_2 (%)	a_3 (%)
Superficial	3	100	—	—	—
Tumorous	8	74	13	—	13
Serrated	152	12	14	44	30
Funnelled	27	7	7	37	48
Spiral	70	4	17	43	36

so deeply (Table VII). The relationship between the type and the depth of invasion was studied in recent cases. All of the superficial type were a_0, many cases of the tumorous type were a_0, and many cases of the funnelled type were a_3, but cases of the spiral type frequently showed a_2 or a_3 invasion (Table VIII).

Operative Methods and End Results

The relationship between operative method and the end result was studied. The end result was better in the cases treated by intrathoracic reconstruction having the cancer in a lower part and with narrow invasion. In the cases of antethoracic reconstruction, the end results of one-step operation were better than the results of divided operation, though only those who had good general and local findings were subjected to the one-step operation. The figures in parentheses in Table IX represent the data obtained from those who received complete reconstruction by the divided operation. Usually, observation was necessary for about 6 months after the resection and, when relapse was not observed during this period, a reconstructive operation was performed. Many cases who could be treated with the second-step reconstructive operation showed retarded development of cancer or complete regression and their end results were as good as those having the one-step operation. The cases whose cancer developed from the thoracic esophagus to the cardia or the gastric body and were treated by esophagojejunostomy showed poor end results, though the number of cases was not so large (Table IX).

TABLE IX.   Operative Methods and 5-Year Survivals (1965-1970)

	No. of cases	No. of 5-year survivals	Crude survival rate (%)
Right thoracic			
Ante-thoracic esophago-gastrostomy	192	36	18.7
Primary reconstructed	53	17	32.0
Divided	139	19	13.6
(Reconstructed)	(27)	(10)	(37.0)
Intrathoracic esophago-gastrostomy	42	12	28.5
Intrathoracic esophago-jejunostomy	2	0	—
Left thoracic esophago-gastrostomy	3	0	—
Total	239	48	20.0

Operative Findings and End Results

Descriptive Rules for Carcinoma of the Esophagus in Clinics and Pathology designate the following items to be described as operative findings: Invasion to adventitia, lymph node metastasis, organ metastasis, pleural dissemination, *etc.* Among these items, invasion to adventitia (a factor) and lymph node metastasis (n factor) will be discussed.

1.   Invasion to adventitia and end results

The rules classify the degree of invasion to adventitia as follows, depending on the histological appearance of the resected specimen:

a_0: no invasion
a_1: possible invasion
a_2: definite invasion
a_3: invasion to a neighboring structure

The end results of the cases of a_2 and a_3 were much worse than those of a_1, and in particular, the 5-year survival was 1.3%, *i.e.*, only 1 case survived among 76 (Table X). The 5-year surviving case was treated with preoperative radiotherapy, but no one survived for more than 2 years after surgery among those of a_3 who were not subjected to preoperative radiotherapy in our clinic.

TABLE X.   Grade of Invasion to Adventitia and 5-Year Survival Rate (1965–1970)

Grade of invasion	No. of cases	No. of 5-year survivals	Crude survival rate (%)
a_0	34	13	38.2
a_1	35	15	42.8
a_2	94	19	20.2
a_3	76	1	1.3

2.   *Lymph node metastasis and end results*

Each lymph node metastasis was recorded following the classification n_0–n_3 by its location, and the cases were classified into 4 groups from Group 1 to Group 4 on the basis for lymph node metastasis. The relationship between the extent of lymph node metastasis and end result is shown in Table XI. The 5-year survival decreased as the n factor increased and it was as low as 8% in n_3 cases (Table XI).

TABLE XI.   Grade of Lymph Node Metastasis and 5-Year Survival Rate (1965–1970)

Grade of lymph node metastasis	No. of cases	No. of 5-year survivals	Crude survival rate (%)
n_0	18	9	50.0
n_1	64	21	32.8
n_2	70	15	21.4
n_3	39	3	7.6

Degree of Progress of Disease and End Results

The degree of progress of the disease was classified into 4 stages from Stage I to Stage IV depending on the degree of maximum invasion to adventitia and lymph

TABLE XII.   Stage of Carcinoma and 5-Year Survival Rate (1965–1970)

Stage	No. of cases	No. of 5-year survivals	Crude survival rate (%)
I	15	6	40.0
II	27	10	37.0
III	94	30	31.9
IV	103	2	1.9

node metastasis, organ metastasis, and pleural dissemination in the operative findings. The end results for the cases of Stage IV were poor (Table XII). There were fewer cases of Stage I and II than of Stage III and IV.

Curability and End Results

The degree of expected cure was classified into 4 degrees from C_0 to C_{III} depending on the progress of carcinoma, resectability of the main lesion, and the degree of removal of the lymph node. A remarkable difference was observed between the prognosis of curative resection groups C_{II} and C_{III} and the noncurative resection groups C_0 and C_I, as shown in Table XIII. The noncurative resection group appeared to include many cases of a_3 and particularly with direct invasion to the bifurcation lymph node (No. 107).

TABLE XIII. Curability and 5-Year Survival Rate (1965–1970)

Grade of curability	No. of cases	No. of 5-year survivals	Crude survival rate (%)
C_{III}–C_{II}	136	44	32.3
C_I–C_0	103	4	3.8

Pathological Classification and End Results

1. Pathological classification of removed specimens

The 5-year survival was 28% in the cases of squamous cell carcinoma of the well-differentiated type and 29% in those of adenocarcinoma, though the number of cases was not large. In the cases of squamous cell carcinoma of the moderately and poorly differentiated types, it was much worse, being 11 to 14% (Table XIV).

TABLE XIV. Pathological Classifications and 5-Year Survival Rate (1965–1970)

Pathological classification	No. of cases	No. of 5-year survivals	Crude survival rate (%)
Squamous cell carcinoma			
Well-differentiated	105	29	27.6
Moderately differentiated	63	7	11.1
Poorly differentiated	22	3	13.6
Adenocarcinoma	7	2	28.5
Carcinoma unclassified	42	7	16.6

2. Vascular invasion and end results

As regards vascular invasion, the end result of 5-year survival was 50% in the ly (−) group (lymphatic invasion absent) while it was 15% in the ly (+) group (lymphatic invasion present). In the v (−) group (blood vessel invasion absent) it was 24%, while it was 12% in the v (+) group (blood vessel invasion present). The difference was not as great as in the ly group (Table XV).

TABLE XV.   Vascular Invasion and 5-Year Survival Rate (1965–1970)

		No. of cases	No. of 5-year survivals	Crude survival rate (%)
Lymphatic invasion	(−)	28	14	50.0
	(+)	188	29	15.4
Not evident		23	5	21.7
Blood vessel invasion	(−)	143	35	24.4
	(+)	68	8	11.7
Not evident		28	5	17.8

Combined Therapy and End Results

I proposed a combined therapy with surgery and radiotherapy in 1958 (5), and some work (1, 9) on combined therapy with preoperative radiotherapy has been reported. Recently, combined therapy with radiotherapy or chemotherapy seems to be the standard treatment for esophageal cancer. In our clinic, most of the recent cases have been treated with preoperative radiation; only particular cases were not subjected to radiotherapy. Therefore, for discussing the end results of combined therapy, the cases treated in Chiba University before 1964 were divided into the concentrated irradiation group, prolonged irradiation group, and non-irradiated group (7).

a)   Thirty-eight cases were exposed to more than 2,500 R in the preoperative radiotherapy, and their 5-year survival was a little better than those exposed to less than 2,499 R. The 5-year survival of the non-irradiated group was 10.9% (Fig. 1).

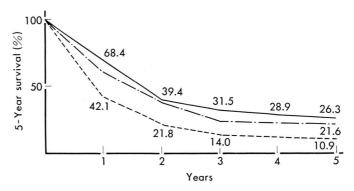

FIG. 1.   Comparative study for 5-year survivals of irradiated or non-irradiated before surgery
——— over 2,500 R irradiated 38 cases; —·— under 2,499 R irradiated 111 cases; – – – – no irradiation 64 cases.

b)   *Relationship between stage of esophageal cancer and preoperative radiotherapy:* The end results were compared between the preoperative radiotherapy group and the non-irradiated group, each group being further classified by the degree of progress of cancer. With any stage of cancer, the end results were better in the irradiated group; particularly, it was interesting that the preoperative radiotherapy was effective in cases with advanced cancer, Stage III and IV (Fig. 2).

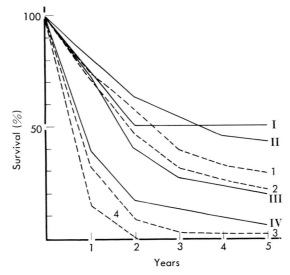

FIG. 2. Relationship between grade of carcinoma of upper and mid-thoracic esophagus and effect of preoperative irradiation

I, 2 cases/4 cases; II, 19/44; III, 8/44; IV, 5/60; 1, 8/28; 2, 21/99; 3, 2/156; 4, 0/59.

Long-term Survival

The 10-year survival of cases with cancer in the upper and middle thoracic esophagus was 9.8% and no large difference was found in those with cancer in the lower esophagocardiac region (Fig. 3).

The number of postoperative long-term surviving patients is stressed in Table XVI (8). The number of patients alive for more than 10 years was 40 when cancer was in the upper and mid-thoracic esophagus and 83 when in the lower esophagus. The number of patients alive for more than 20 years was 4 with cancer in the upper and mid-thoracic esophagus and 5 in the lower esophagus.

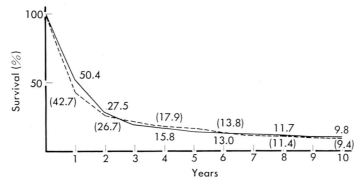

FIG. 3. Postoperative long-term survival rate following operation for carcinoma of esophagus

——— carcinoma of upper and mid-thoracic esophagus; – – – – carcinoma of lower esophagus and gastric cardia.

TABLE XVI. Number of Postoperative Long-term Survivals for Carcinoma
of the Esophagus (1945–1974, Nakayama)

	Over 5 years (cases)	Over 10 years (cases)	Over 15 years (cases)	Over 20 years (cases)
Upper and mid-thoracic esophagus	110	40	13	4
Lower esophagus and gastric cardia	199	83	30	5
Total	309	123	43	9

Esophageal cancer cannot be completely cured by improvement of the operational technique alone (12). The development of a combined therapy with radiation or anti-cancer chemotherapy and immunotherapy is required. Furthermore, an essential challenge to the disease "cancer" itself is required, and this is the real problem for the future.

REFERENCES

1. Akakura, I. and Shimamura, Y. Cancer of the esophagus. *Kyobu Geka* (*Japan. J. Thorac. Surg.*), **21**, 247–253 (1968) (in Japanese).
2. Endo, M., Hanyu, F., Kinoshita, Y., Ide, H., and Nakayama, K. Post-operative survivals of the thoracic esophageal cancer. *Surgical Diagnosis and Treatment* (*Geka Shinryo*), **18**, 863–867 (1976) (in Japanese).
3. Japanese Society for Esophageal Diseases. "Guide Lines for the Clinical and Pathological Studies on Carcinoma of the Esophagus," Kanehara Shuppan, Tokyo (1969).
4. Kobayashi, S. The study of the preoperative irradiation therapy for the upper and mid thoracic esophageal cancer. *Nippon Kyobu Geka Gakkai Zasshi* (*J. Japan. Assoc. Thorac. Surg.*), **12**, 625–677 (1964) (in Japanese).
5. Nakayama, K., Yanagisawa, F., Nabeya, K., Tamiya, T., Kobayashi, S., and Makino, K. Concentrated preoperative irradiation therapy. *Arch. Surg.*, **87**, 1003–1018 (1963).
6. Nakayama, K., Nabeya, K., Makino, K., and Hoshino, K. Evaluation of patients living more than five years after operation. *Rinsho Geka* (*J. Clin. Surg.*), **20**, 1033–1039 (1966) (in Japanese).
7. Nakayama, K. and Kinoshita, Y. Surgical treatment combined with preoperative concentrated irradiation. *J. Am. Med. Assoc.*, **227**, 178–181 (1974).
8. Nakayama, K., Kinoshita, Y., Endo, M., Ide, H., and Momma, K. Treatment and survival results of esophageal carcinoma. *Nihon-rinsho* (*Japan. J. Clin. Med.*), **378**, 880–891 (1974) (in Japanese).
9. Parker, E. F. and Gregorie, H. B., Jr. Combined radiation and surgical treatment of carcinoma of the esophagus. *Ann. Surg.*, **16**, 710–718 (1965).
10. Sato, H., Sato, F., Isono, K., Koike, Y., Onoda, S., Okuyama, K., Saito, T., Karashi, N., and Yamamoto, Y. Surgical results of esophageal carcinoma. *Shijutsu* (*Operation*), **32**, 153–159 (1978) (in Japanese).
11. Seo, S. Surgery of the esophagus. *Nippon Geka Gakkai Zasshi* (*J. Japan. Surg. Soc.*), **33**, 1461–1505 (1932) (in Japanese).
12. Young Husband, J. D. and Aluwihare, A.P.R. Carcinoma of the oesophagus; factors influencing survival. *Br. J. Surg.*, **57**, 422–430 (1970).

CANCER OF THE LUNG IN JAPAN

Yoshihiro Hayata and Hideo Funatsu

*Department of Surgery, Tokyo Medical College**

Postoperative results were compared between resection-only cases and combined therapy cases in 1,414 resected cases out of a total of 3,345 lung cancer cases which were treated by the Hayata Research Project Group of the Ministry of Health and Welfare from 1962 to 1970. The 5-year survival rate was 28% for all resected cases, 67.5% for Stage I, 36.7% for Stage II, and 13.5% for Stage III. Comparison of the relationship between the 5-year survival rate and therapeutic method according to histological type showed that in Stage I the best results were obtained in resection-only squamous cell carcinoma and adeno-carcinoma cases, but in large cell carcinoma the best result was obtained in irradiation plus chemotherapy cases. In Stage II, the best results were obtained in chemotherapy cases with resection for all histological types. In Stage III, the best results were obtained in irradiation plus chemotherapy in squamous cell carcinoma and large cell carcinoma, whereas chemotherapy achieved the best results for adenocarcinoma. Break-down of the results according to the main Stage III classification factors in cases of lymph node metastasis in the mediastinum and chest wall invasion showed that the best result was obtained by irradiation plus chemotherapy with resection, while the best result was obtained by chemotherapy in pleural invasion cases. Thus, combined therapy with resection for lung cancer should be selected after many factors have been examined, including histological type and clinical stages.

During the past decade various types of adjuvant therapies have been utilized to improve the prognosis of lung cancer cases, and since 1971 the Hayata Research Project Group of the Ministry of Health and Welfare has been examining and evaluating the therapeutic methods in lung cancer cases, based on past results using data from histology, clinical stage, cell features of the tumor cells, and histogenesis. This group consists of Department of Surgery and Roentgenology of Tokyo Medical College, Department of Internal Medicine of Dokkyo Medical School, Department of Pathology of Keio University, Lung Cancer Institute of Chiba University, Research Institute for Tuberculosis, Leprosy, and Cancer of Tohoku University, Thoracic Surgery Division of Center for Adult Diseases, Osaka, Thoracic Surgery Division and Pathology Division of Kyushu Cancer Center, Surgery Division of Nakano National Hospital, and Department of Surgery of Cancer Institute Hospital, Tokyo.

A total of 3,345 cases of lung cancer were treated at these institutes from 1962 until 1970 and ages ranged from 19 to 82 years, averaging 59.7 years. The male-to-female ratio was 5.5: 1. Of these 3,345 cases, 1,414 underwent resection and, histologi-

* Nishishinjuku 6-7-1, Shinjuku-ku, Tokyo 160, Japan (早田義博, 船津秀夫).

cally, 44.9% of these were squamous cell carcinoma, 33.1% adenocarcinoma, 16.2% large cell carcinoma, while only 5.8% of the resected cases were small cell carcinoma. Owing to the small number of small cell carcinoma cases they have been excluded from the present series. Only 42 (22.5%) of 186 small cell carcinoma cases were resected and only 3 cases survived 5 years or more.

The postoperative results will be presented by comparing therapeutic methods such as resection alone and resection plus irradiation and/or chemotherapy according to histological type. These resected cases were clinically and surgically staged according to the TNM classification of the American Joint Committee. Of the cases resected up to the end of 1959, resection-only cases constituted 75.0%, the remaining 25.0% also receiving adjuvant therapy. In those treated after 1960, resection-only cases dropped to 11.9% and the remaining 88.1% were treated with irradiation or chemotherapy pre- or post-operatively. Therefore, it can be said that the results of resection-only cases are primarily those of cases treated up to 1959 while combined therapy cases are those cases treated after 1960.

Results of Treatments

The relationship between resectability and 5-year survival rates according to clinical stages by the TNM classification is shown in Table I, the best resectability and 5-year survival rate being obtained in Stage I cases, followed by Stage II and III. The 5-year survival rate was 67.5% in Stage I, 36.7% in Stage II, and 13.5% in Stage III. The difference was statistically significant ($\chi^2 = 185.7$, DF$=2$; $p < 0.001$). The results of combined therapy with resection were compared with those of resection-only cases (Table II). The best 5-year survival rate was 76.8% in Stage I cases with

TABLE I. Relationship between Resectability and 5-Year Survival
Rates According to Clinical Stage

Stage	No. of cases	Resectability (%)	5-Year relative survival rate	
			No. of cases	%
I	355	90.7	270	67.5
II	410	82.1	306	36.7
III	2,580	29.4	586	13.5

$\chi^2 = 185.75$, DF$=2$, $p < 0.001$.

TABLE II. Relationship between Combined Therapy and 5-Year
Survival Rates According to Clinical Stage

Stage	Resection-only		Resection with					
			Irradiation		Chemotherapy		Irradiation+ chemotherapy	
	Cases	%	Cases	%	Cases	%	Cases	%
I	79	76.8	54	63.6	99	61.3	38	69.3
II	68	26.9	70	31.1	98	52.6	56	30.7
III	56	13.0	159	14.4	184	16.8	128	18.8

resection alone, however, the difference was not statistically significant ($\chi^2 = 3.72$, DF = 3; $p < 0.9$). In Stage II cases, the best result was obtained in chemotherapy cases with resection (52.6%), and in Stage III cases the best result was obtained in cases which received irradiation plus chemotherapy (18.8%). The differences were statistically significant ($\chi^2 = 12.27$, DF = 3; $p < 0.01$, and $\chi^2 = 7.75$, DF = 3; $p < 0.01$, respectively). Many kinds of combined therapeutic methods were used in this series such as pre- or post-operative irradiation with or without chemotherapy, and chemotherapy with a single drug or with multiple drug combinations (Fig. 1). Possible combinations of therapeutic methods are shown in Fig. 2. Five-year survival rates in terms of clinical stage and histological type were compared between resection-only cases and combined therapy cases receiving surgical operation. In Stage I cases the best results were ob-

Irradiation

a. Preoperative irradiation

b. Postoperative irradiation

Chemotherapy (pre-or postoperatively)

a. Single drug methods

MMC	2 mg every day, i.v. or orally or 4–6 mg twice a week, i.v.
Chromomycin	0.5 mg every day, i.v.
Cyclophosphamide	100 mg every day i.v. or orally or 1000 mg once a week, i.v.
BLM	15–30 mg twice a week, i.v.

b. Multiple combination methods

METT ; MMC 2 mg
Cyclophosphamide 100 mg
Chromomycin 0.5 mg
Thio-TEPA 10 mg
One drug each day in turn by i.v. × 8 times = 32 days

FAMT ; 5-Fluorouracil 250 mg
Cyclophosphamide 100 mg
MMC 2 mg
Chromomycin 0.5 mg
One drug each day in turn by i.v. × 8 days = 32 days

Intervals between therapeutic courses of METT and FAMT vary, depending on patient's condition etc.

c. Intermittent administration

Chromomycin 0.5 mg
MMC 2.0 mg
every day × 30 days, once every 4–6 months

Every day for one month of a 6-month or 4-month therapeutic period. Nothing else administered for remainder of period. Long-term regular intermittent therapy.

d. Three-drug administration

5-FU 250 mg
MMC 2 mg
Cyclophosphamide 100 mg
One drug each day in turn – long term

FIG. 1. Combined therapy methods with resection (Hayata Group)

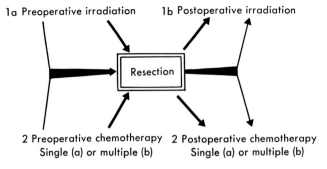

FIG. 2.   Possible combination of therapeutic methods

tained in resection-only squamous cell carcinoma (84.5%) and adenocarcinoma (74.1%), but in large cell carcinoma the best result was obtained by irradiation plus chemotherapy (69.3%). However, the difference between resection-only cases and combined therapy cases was not statistically significant ($\chi^2=3.19$, DF$=2$; $p<0.1$) (Table III). Similarly, the 5-year survival rates were compared in relation to histological type and combined therapy in Stage II cases (Table IV). Regardless of the histological type, the best result was obtained in cases which received chemotherapy with resection; 51.7% in squamous cell carcinoma, 37.4% in adenocarcinoma, and 53.4% in large cell carcinoma. However, the difference between resection-only cases and combined therapy cases was not

TABLE III.   Relationship between 5-Year Relative Survival Rates and Combined Therapy According to Histological Type in Stage I Resected Cases

| | Resection-only | | Resection with | | | | | |
| | | | Irradiation | | Chemotherapy | | Irradiation+ chemotherapy | |
	Cases	%	Cases	%	Cases	%	Cases	%
Squamous cell carcinoma	42	84.5	24	71.5	50	66.4	13	70.5
Adenocarcinoma	17	74.1	15	53.5	23	59.8	17	67.4
Large cell carcinoma	20	63.0	15	61.1	26	52.9	8	71.6
Total	79	76.8	54	63.6	99	61.3	38	69.3

TABLE IV.   Relationship between 5-Year Relative Survival Rates and Combined Therapy According to Histological Type in Stage II Resected Cases

| | Resection-only | | Resection with | | | | | |
| | | | Irradiation | | Chemotherapy | | Irradiation+ chemotherapy | |
	Cases	%	Cases	%	Cases	%	Cases	%
Squamous cell carcinoma	35	39.3	29	47.4	51	51.7	23	39.8
Adenocarcinoma	19	12.1	26	17.6	46	37.4	20	22.9
Large cell carcinoma	14	16.4	15	22.9	15	53.4	13	17.6
Total	68	26.9	Total combined therapy		224 cases		39.8%	

TABLE V. Relationship between 5-Year Relative Survival Rates and Combined Therapy According to Histological Type in Stage III Resected Cases

| | Resection-only | | Resection with | | | | | |
| | | | Irradiation | | Chemotherapy | | Irradiation+ chemotherapy | |
	Cases	%	Cases	%	Cases	%	Cases	%
Squamous cell carcinoma	29	11.8	79	20.3	91	18,8	59	21.3
Adenocarcinoma	10	0	54	4.2	70	18.0	47	14.6
Large cell carcinoma	8	0	26	17.6	23	4.9	22	20.8
Total	56	6.1	Total combined therapy		471 cases		15.0%	

statistically significant for all histological types ($\chi^2=5.62$, DF$=3$; $p<0.9$; $\chi^2=5.09$, DF$=3$; $p<0.5$; and $\chi^2=5.62$, DF$=3$; $p<0.5$, respectively). In Stage III cases (Table V) of squamous cell carcinoma and large cell carcinoma, the best results were obtained in cases which received chemotherapy and irradiation with resection, 21.3% and 20.8%, respectively, while in adenocarcinoma the best result (18.0%) was achieved in chemotherapy cases with resection. The difference was not statistically significant in squamous cell carcinoma or large cell carcinoma ($\chi^2=1.05$, DF$=3$; $p<0.5$, and $\chi^2=3.57$, DF$=3$; $0.1>p$, respectively) and the statistical difference was moderate in adenocarcinoma ($\chi^2=7.42$, DF$=3$; $0.05>p$). In the data for all Stage III cases, many factors are included, regardless of the factor which caused them to be classified as such, *e.g.*, effusion, lymph node metastasis in the supraclavicular region, Pancoast tumor, *etc*. However, cases having these factors are very few, therefore the effect of combined therapy with resection was analyzed by breaking down the Stage III classification factors as shown in Table VI. The best 5-year survival rate was obtained with irradiation plus chemotherapy with resection (15.9%) in cases of lymph node metastasis in the mediastinum and chest wall invasion (28.6%), while in pleural invasion cases, the best 5-year survival rate was in chemotherapy cases (20.0%). The difference was not statistically significant for all factors ($\chi^2=2.67$, DF$=3$; $p<0.9$, $\chi^2=3.55$, DF$=3$; $p<0.5$, and $\chi^2=0.749$, DF$=3$; $p<0.9$, respectively). Observation of the effect of preoperative irradiation in Stage II and III cases (Table VII) showed that the best result was obtained in preoperative irradiation in Stage III (17.4%) but not in Stage II cases. The difference was statistically significant compared with Stage II chemotherapy cases ($\chi^2=9.38$;

TABLE VI. Relationship between 5-Year Relative Survival Rates and Combined Therapy According to Main Stage III Classification Factors

| | Resection-only | | Resection with | | | | | |
| | | | Irradiation | | Chemotherapy | | Irradiation+ chemotherapy | |
	Cases	%	Cases	%	Cases	%	Cases	%
Lymph node metastasis in mediastinum	32	3.6	78	11.7	77	14.9	43	15.9
Pleural invasion	4	0	24	9.5	40	20.0	38	18.1
Chest wall invasion	19	18.8	49	21.0	27	21.2	16	28.6

TABLE VII. Therapeutic Efficacy in Terms of 5-Year Relative Survival Rates

Treatment	Stage II		Stage III	
	Cases	%	Cases	%
Resection only	68	26.9	56	6.1
Resection with chemotherapy	98	49.1	184	17.4
Preoperative irradiation	51	33.7	96	17.9
Other combined therapy	57	50.2	191	15.0

DF$=3$; $p<0.01$), however the difference was not statistically significant for all the factors in Stage III cases ($\chi^2=3.988$, DF$=3$; $p<0.1$).

DISCUSSION

The postresection 5-year survival rates in lung cancer cases ranges between 17.3% and 29% in recent reports (1, 3, 8, 11, 18), and that of the Hayata Research Project Group was 28%. With regard to factors which control postoperative prognosis, there has been much discussion about the relationship to histological type, location of the tumor, clinical stage, presence or absence of lymph node metastasis, and invasion into adjacent tissues or organs, extent of resection, and the use of combined therapy with resection. There are many reports concerning adjuvant therapies with resection. Chemotherapy with surgery is the most common method at present for lung cancer cases, and improved results have been reported by Katuki (8), Brunner (2), and others by long-term administration of cyclophosphamide, mitomycin C (MMC) or chromomycin, and better results were reported in small cell carcinoma by administering cyclophosphamide, vincristine, or bleomycin (BLM) by Horai (7), Einhorn (5), and others (12). Additionally, in Japan, recent chemotherapeutic methods include multicombination methods such as METT, FAMT (13) (Fig. 1), with or without surgery. In our series, better results were obtained in Stage II cases receiving chemotherapy with resection compared to resection-only cases, although this was not so in Stage I and III cases. Recently, I have been administering anticancer agents in different combinations according to histological type as follows: In squamous cell carcinoma three drugs, cyclophosphamide, chromomycin, and BLM; in adenocarcinoma, 3 drugs, 5-fluorouracil (5-FU), MMC, and chromomycin; and in small cell carcinoma 4 drugs, cyclophosphamide, vincristine, chromomycin, and BLM. By the use of histological type-based chemotherapeutic methods, slightly better results were obtained in squamous cell carcinoma and in small cell carcinoma as compared with the old method which ignored the histological type. Selection of the methods relied on basic research examining the sensitivity of cultured cells, established from human lung cancer cases, to various drugs. In irradiation therapy with resection, postoperative irradiation was employed in Stage II and III cases with lymph node metastasis or invasion and as reported Martini (9), in our cases better results were obtained in Stage II cases of squamous cell carcinoma and large cell carcinoma compared to resection-only cases, but it was not effective in Stage II adenocarcinoma cases. Furthermore, in Stage III cases better results were obtained in irradiated cases compared to resection-only cases. Green (6) reported that better results were obtained in cases with metastasis to the lymph nodes of the hilum or mediastinum compared to nonmetastatic cases, whereas in our series 5-year survival for cases of chest wall invasion without metastasis was significantly higher than that for mediastinal lymph node metastasis. Reports concerning preoperative irradiation have also been made by Shields (14), Warram (17), and others. To sum up, our data concerning preoperative irradiation, it is possible to say that heretofore better results have been obtained than in resection-only cases in Stages II and III, but not compared to chemotherapy, the latter results of which also do not seem to be improved by use in conjunction with irradiation, except, perhaps, when examined in terms of Stage I 5-year survival. Generally, preoperative irradiation is not indicated as a routine method for all stages of lung cancer, and, in our experience, better results were not always obtained in Stage III cases compared to those of chemotherapy, but remarkable improvement was obtained compared to resection-only cases of mediastinal lymph node metastasis and pleural invasion cases. However, according to the results of preoperative irradiation at the Department of Surgery, Tokyo Medical College, cases surviving 5 years or more, with metastasis to the lymph nodes of the mediastinum and/or invasion into the chest wall were included among those cases which received preoperative irradiation in squamous cell carcinoma. There was no such case surviving 5 years or more which had been treated even by other combined therapy in adenocarcinoma. Therefore, preoperative irradiation should be performed in these cases. In irradiation plus chemotherapy cases with resection, better results were obtained in Stage III of squamous cell carcinoma and large cell carcinoma, but there was no effect in adenocarcinoma, nor in Stage I and II cases including squamous cell carcinoma, adenocarcinoma, and large cell carcinoma. Thus, for the present, it may be thought that combined therapy with resection should be performed as follows: T_1n_0 Stage I; no adjuvant therapy at all; T_1n_1 Stage I cases; chemotherapy or chemotherapy with immunotherapy; Stage II cases of squamous cell carcinoma and large cell carcinoma, chemotherapy plus irradiation or immunotherapy; Stage II adenocarcinoma cases chemotherapy or chemotherapy plus immunotherapy; Stage III cases of squamous cell carcinoma and large cell carcinoma, chemotherapy plus irradiation plus/or immunotherapy, especially preoperative irradiation for chest wall invasion or mediastinal lymph node metastasis cases, Stage III adenocarcinoma; chemotherapy plus immunotherapy or postoperative irradiation. Immunotherapy as an adjuvant therapy is mentioned above. Recently, many reports concerning immunotherapy in lung cancer have been made by Edwards and Whitwell (4), Swierenga et al. (16), McKneally et al. (10), and others, however, it is too early to fully estimate the effect of immunotherapy on lung cancer yet. In Japan, immunotherapy for lung cancer has been conducted using BCG or BCG-cell wall skeleton (CWS) by Yamamura's group at the Department of Internal Medicine, Osaka University, among others. I have been investigating the immunoresponse of lung cancer cases by examining T-cell population changes, blast formation by phytohemagglutinin, and colony inhibition tests with cultured cells and lymphocytes; the existence of immuneresponse in some cases of lung cancer, even in Stage III, was demonstrated, therefore lung cancer cases are treated immunologically by intrapleural cavity, subcutaneous, intrabronchial, or intratumor injection of BCG or BCG-CWS. However, the results cannot be discussed since only a short period has elapsed since the commencement of this method.

Finally, I feel that combined therapy used with resection in lung cancer should be selected after many factors have been taken into account in order to obtain maximum effectiveness.

Acknowledgment

This work was supported by a Grant-in-Aid for Cancer Research from the Ministry of Health and Welfare, Japan.

REFERENCES

1. Ashor, G. L., Kern, W. H., Mayer, B. W., Lindesmith, G. G., Stiles, Q. R., Tucker, B. L., and Jones, J. Long-term survival in bronchogenic carcinoma. *J. Thorac. Cardiovasc. Surg.*, **70**, 581–859 (1975).
2. Brunner, K. W., Marthaler, T., and Müller, W. Effects of long-term adjuvant chemotherapy with cyclophosphamide for radically resected bronchogenic carcinoma. *Cancer Chemother. Rep.* Part 3., **4**, 125–130 (1973).
3. Debesse, B., Priollet, D., Grenier, G., Dubost, Cl., and Thomeret, G. Cancer primitif bronchique opéré. Étude de la survie chez 560 malades. *Nouv. Presse Méd.*, **4**, 2639–2642 (1975).
4. Edwards, F. R. and Whitwell, F. Use of BCG as an immunostimulant in the surgical treatment of carcinoma of the lung. *Thorax*, **29**, 654–658 (1974).
5. Einhorn, L. H., Fee, W. H., Faber, M. O., Livingston, R. B., and Gottlieb, J. A. Improved chemotherapy for small-cell undifferentiated lung cancer. *J. Am. Med. Assoc.*, **235**, 1225–1229 (1976).
6. Green, N., Kurohara, S. S., George, F. W., and Crews, Q. E. Postresection irradiation for primary lung cancer. *Radiology*, **116**, 405–407 (1975).
7. Horai, T., Matsuda, M., Ikegami, H., Takenaga, A., and Hattori, S. On the intermittent large dose administration of cyclophosphamide for small cell carcinoma of the lung. *Gan-to-Kagakuryoho* (*Cancer Chemother.*), **3**, 41 (1976) (in Japanese).
8. Katuki, H., Shimada, K., Koyama, A., Okita, M., Yamaguchi, Y., Okamoto T., and Benfield, J. R. Long-term intermittent adjuvant chemotherapy for primary, resected lung cancer. *J. Thorac. Cardiovasc. Surg.*, **70**, 590–599 (1975).
9. Martini, N., Hilaris, B. S., and Beattie, E. J. Interstitial *vs.* external irradiation combined with pulmonary resection in lung cancer. *Cancer*, **26**, 638–641 (1970).
10. McKneally, M. F., Maver, C., and Kausel, H. W. Regional immunotherapy of lung cancer with intrapleural B.C.G. *Lancet*, **i**, 377–379 (1976).
11. Naruke, T., Suemasu, K., and Ishikawa, S. Surgical treatment for lung cancer with metastasis to mediastinal lymph nodes. *J. Thorac. Cardiovasc. Surg.*, **71**, 281–289 (1976).
12. Niitani, H. Chemotherapy of lung cancer. *Gan-to-Kagakuryoho* (*Cancer Chemother.*), **3**, 50–58 (1976) (in Japanese).
13. Nishimura, M. Combination chemotherapy for lung cancer. *Gan-to-Kagakuryoho* (*Cancer Chemother.*), **3**, 34–39 (1976) (in Japanese).
14. Shields, T. W., Higgins, G. A., Lawton, R., Heilbrum, A., and Keehn, R. J. Preoperative X-ray therapy as an adjuvant in the treatment of bronchogenic carcinoma. *J. Thorac. Cardiovasc. Surg.*, **59**, 49–62 (1970).
15. Stoloff, I. L. The prognostic value of bronchoscopy in primary lung cancer. *J. Am. Med. Assoc.*, **227**, 299–301 (1974).
16. Swierenga, J., Gooszen, H. C., Vanderschueren, R. G., Cosemans, J., Louwagie, A., Stam, J., Veldhuigen, R. W., Cardozo, E. L., Ceuster, G. D., Tanghe, W., Janseen, P.A.J., Drochmans, A., Dony, J., Desplenter, L., Denissen, E., and Ammeery, W.

Immunopotentiation with levamisol in resectable bronchogenic carcinoma. A double-blind controlled trial. *Br. Med. J.*, **3**, 461–464 (1975).

17. Warram, J. Preoperative irradiation of cancer of the lung. Final report of a therapeutic trial. *Cancer*, **36**, 914–925 (1975).
18. Vincent, R. G., Takita, H., Lane, W. W., Gutierrez, A. C., and Pickren, J. W. Surgical therapy of lung cancer. *J. Thorac. Cardiovasc. Surg.*, **71**, 581–591 (1976).

CANCER OF THE LUNG AT THE NATIONAL CANCER CENTER, TOKYO

Shichiro Ishikawa, Keiichi Suemasu, Toshiro Ogata,
Takeshi Yoneyama, Tsuguo Naruke, and
Yukio Shimosato

*Pathology Division, Department of Surgery,
National Cancer Center Hospital**

At the National Cancer Center, Tokyo, 1,035 cases with lung cancer were treated in the 9-year period from 1962 to 1971; 412 underwent pulmonary resection. The sex ratio was approximately 4 males to 1 female. The age distribution showed the highest incidence in the sixties. A reasonable relationship between postsurgical histopathological TNM staging and survival was established, *i.e.*, the relative 5-year survival rate was 69.4% in Stage I, 38.7% in Stage II, and 9.0% in Stage III. The relationship of cell type to prognosis was reaffirmed. Squamous cell carcinoma was associated with the best chance of survival, whereas small cell carcinoma did worst. In evaluating treatment modalities such as resection, radiation, or chemotherapy, it may be necessary to subclassify small cell carcinoma into the oat cell type and intermediate cell type. The latter showed a better prognosis following pulmonary resection. The degree of operative curability, lymph node status, and extent of pleural invasion have all been found to correlate well with the 5-year survival rate.

Staging and histological classification of lung cancer have been subjected to a great deal of world-wide discussion. This has led to a fair degree of agreement in classification and criteria, which can readily be adopted in many countries. Nevertheless, there appears to be an obvious need for further modification and standardization.

In this report, the clinical and pathological features of 412 patients with lung cancer treated by pulmonary resection at the National Cancer Center Hospital are reviewed. The study was conducted to determine prognosis after surgical resection.

Clinical Materials, Classifications for Extent of Disease, and Histology

One thousand and thirty-five patients with lung cancer were treated at the National Cancer Center Hospital in the 9-year period from May, 1962 to May, 1971. Thoracotomy was performed on 491 patients (47.4%), including 412 resections and 79 exploratory thoracotomies. The rate of nonresectability among the patients subjected to thoracotomy was 16.0% (Table I). None of the patients was lost to follow-up study.

Staging was performed according to the postsurgical histopathological TNM system which was our criteria, followed by histopathological examination of resected

---

* Tsukiji 5-1-1, Chuo-ku, Tokyo 104, Japan (石川七郎, 末舛恵一, 尾形利郎, 米山武志, 成毛韶夫, 下里幸雄).

TABLE I. Modality of Surgical Treatment in Patients with Lung Cancer

	No. of cases
Hospitalized	1,035
Treated	1,014
Thoracotomized	491
Exploratory	79
Resectional	412
Curative	153
Relatively curative	102
Noncurative	157

(NCCH, Tokyo (1962–1971)).

specimens applying existing clinical TNM system (15). The staging was supplemented by applying the surgical-pathological classification of the Japan Lung Cancer Society (JLCS) relating to pleural invasion and lymph node metastasis (5).

The categorization with regard to the extent of disease to the lymph nodes, verified by microscopic examination, is as follows:

n_0: No involved lymph nodes.

n_1: Positive nodes only in the intrapulmonary location.

n_2: Positive nodes up to the hilum.

n_3: Positive nodes in the mediastinum.

n_4: Positive nodes in the supraclavicular location.

The categorization with regard to the extent of invasion to the pleura and neighboring structures determined histologically is as follows:

p_0: Tumor present apart from the pleura.

p_1: Tumor reaching the visceral pleura, but not extending beyond its elastic layer.

p_2: Tumor involving the visceral pleura, but not the neighboring structures.

p_3: Tumor infiltrating in continuity the neighboring structures, *e.g.*, parietal pleura, chest wall, *etc.*, or disseminating in the pleural cavity.

Surgical treatment in each patient was designated depending on the degree of its curability as curative, relatively curative, or noncurative resection. The criteria established by the JLCS were used for this categorization (5). Curative resections are those in which the tumor is grossly and microscopically confined within the resected lung, pleura ($p \leq 1$), and bronchus with no mediastinal or carinal lymph node involvement ($n \leq 2$), and when an *en bloc* pulmonary resection with mediastinal dissection is performed. Many of the pulmonary resections performed for clinical Stage I and II disease are categorized in this group. Relatively curative resections are those in which the tumor has grown beyond the visceral pleura ($p \geq 2$) and/or positive mediastinal lymph nodes are present ($n = 3$), and when an *en bloc* complete resection is thought to have been accomplished. Pulmonary resections for clinical Stage III disease without distant metastases (M_0) are often categorized in this group. Noncurative resections are defined as the situation where obvious residual disease is present or strongly suspected. Stage III cases usually constitute this group.

Histological classification of the tumors was made according to the criteria of the

National Cancer Center Hospital (NCCH) (6) which is a slight modification of the classification of the World Health Organization (WHO) (9).

Relative 5-Year Survival Rates of Resected Lung Cancer Cases

The age and sex data of the 412 cases are summarized in Table II. The male-to-female ratio was 3.6 to 1. When sex was correlated with age distribution, the highest sex ratio, that is 5: 1, was observed in the sixties. The age distribution showed the highest peak in the sixties, which seemed to represent the high incidence of the disease in males in this age group. In females, however, the disease is relatively more common in a younger age group with a somewhat widened peak of distribution between the age of 50 and 69 years.

One hundred and twelve patients (including 7 cases of lung cancer with low-grade malignancy) survived for 5 years or longer after pulmonary resection. These 112 patients surviving longer than 5 years represented 10.8% of the entire group of 1,035 hospitalized patients.

The 412 resected cases were classified by the histopathological TNM staging system and the staging was compared with survival data. Number of patients at each stage was: Stage I—137 (33.3%); Stage II—45 (10.9%); and Stage III—230 (55.8%) (Table III). The relative 5-year survival rates of operative survivors in these groups were: Stage I—69.4% (74/129); Stage II—38.8% (15/44); and Stage III—9.0% (16/208) (Table IV).

Histological classification of 412 resected cases was then made according to the

TABLE II. Sex and Age Incidence of Lung Cancer

Age (years)	No. of cases		
	Males	Females	Total
–39	15	6	21
40–49	40	15	55
50–59	95	31	126
60–69	142	28	170
70–	30	10	40
Total	322	90	412

(NCCH, Tokyo (1962–1971)).

TABLE III. Stage of Disease in 412 Patients with Lung Cancer who Underwent Resection

Stage	Patients	
	Number	%
I	137 (5)	33.3
II	45	10.9
III	230 (2)	55.8

Figures in parentheses indicate the number of cases with low-grade malignant cancer.
(NCCH, Tokyo (1962–1971)).

TABLE IV. Survival of Patients Following Resection of Lung Cancer:
Relative 5-Year Survival Rate by Stage

Stage	No. of patients[a]	No. of operative deaths	5-Year survival rate[b] (%)
I	132	3	69.4*
II	45	1	38.8*
III	228	20	9.0*
Total	405	24	32.2 ± 2.4[c]

* $p < 0.05$.
[a] Excluding cases of low-grade malignant cancer.
[b] Excluding cases of early postoperative death.
[c] Standard error.
(NCCH, Tokyo (1962–1971)).

TABLE V. Survival of Patients Following Resection of Lung Cancer: Relative
5-Year Survival Rate by Cell Type

Cell type	Patients		No. of operative deaths	5-Year survival rate[a] (%)
	Number	%		
Squamous cell	152	36.9	8	43.3*
Small cell	25	6.1	3	15.4*
Adenocarcinoma	170	41.3	9	27.7*
Large cell	35	8.5	3	33.7
Others	23	5.6	1	44.0
Total	405		24	32.2 ± 2.4
Carcinoma of low malignancy	7	1.7	0	102.5

* $p < 0.05$.
[a] Excluding cases of early postoperative death.
(NCCH, Tokyo (1962–1971)).

NCCH criteria and was compared with survival data (Table V). Number of cases in each histological type was: Squamous cell carcinomas 152 (36.9%); small cell carcinomas 25 (6.1%); adenocarcinomas 170 (41.3%); large cell carcinomas 35 (8.5%); carcinomas of low-grade malignancy 7 (1.7%); others 23 (5.6%) (17 with adenosquamous and 8 with unclassified cell type). The relative 5-year survival rates of operative survivors in these histological cell types were: Squamous cell carcinomas 43.3% (52/144); small cell carcinomas 15.4% (3/22); adenocarcinomas 27.7% (33/161); large cell carcinomas 33.7% (9/32); others 44.0% (9/22), and carcinomas of low-grade malignancy 102.5% (7/7).

Pulmonary resections performed in 405 patients were categorized into 3 groups depending on the degree of curability, and the survival data were then analyzed in each category (Table VI). Patients with low-grade malignant carcinoma were excluded from the survival data. Number of cases in these categories were: Curative resections 147 (36.2%); relatively curative resections 102 (25.2%) and noncurative resections 156 (38.5%). The relative 5-year survival rates of operative survivors in these categories were: Curative resections 67.4% (81/142); relatively curative resections 21.5% (18/97); noncurative resections 4.9% (6/142).

TABLE VI. Survival of Patients Following Resection of Lung Cancer: Relative 5-Year Survival Rate by Degree of Operative Curability

Degree of operative curability	No. of cases[a]	No. of operative deaths	5-Year survival rate[b] (%)
Curative	147	5	67.4*
Relatively curative	102	5	21.5
Noncurative	156	14	4.9*
Total	405	24	32.2±2.4

* $p < 0.05$.

[a] Excluding cases of low-grade malignant cancer.

[b] Excluding cases of early postoperative death.

(NCCH, Tokyo (1962–1971)).

TABLE VII. Survival of Patients Following Resection of Lung Cancer: Relative 5-Year Survival Rate by Lymph Node Status

	No. of cases[a]	No. of operative deaths	5-Year survival rate[b] (%)
n_0	147	5	57.2*
n_1	14	0	68.0*
n_2	71	3	37.1*
n_3	140	13	7.2
n_4	33	3	0
Total	405	24	32.2±2.4

* Significant compared with n_3 and n_4 groups ($p < 0.05$).

[a] Excluding cases of low-grade malignant cancer.

[b] Excluding cases of early postoperative death.

(NCCH, Tokyo (1962–1971)).

Microscopic examinations were made on the intrapulmonary, interlobar, hilar, and mediastinal lymph nodes dissected at the time of and after surgery. The lymph node status was then compared with prognosis (Table VII). Among the 405 patients, there were 147 cases (36.3%) without lymph node metastasis (n_0). Fourteen cases (3.4%) showed the disease in the intrapulmonary node(s) (n_1). Seventy-one cases (17.5%) had metastatic disease in the interlobar and/or hilar lymph node(s) (n_2). The mediastinal lymph node(s) was involved with metastasis in 140 cases (34.6%) (n_3), and there was positive supraclavicular lymph node(s) in 33 cases (8.1%) (n_4). The relative 5-year survival rates of operative survivors according to lymph node status were: n_0—57.2% (67/142); n_1—68.0% (8/14); n_2—37.1% (22/68); n_3—7.2% (8/127); and n_4—0% (0/30).

The 405 resected cases were then divided into 4 categories according to the status of pleural invasion of the disease and 5-year survival was studied (Table VIII). Tumors of low-grade malignancy were again excluded from the survival data.

There were 105 patients (25.9%) whose tumor had not reached the visceral pleura (p_0). The relative 5-year survival rates among the operative survivors with p_0 disease was 46.0% (39/99). In 134 patients (33.1%) the tumor had reached the visceral pleura (p_1) and the survival rate was 46.0% (50/127). In 93 patients (22.9%) the tumor had

TABLE VIII. Survival of Patients Following Resection of Lung Cancer: Relative 5-Year Survival Rate by Degree of Pleural Involvement

	No. of cases[a]	No. of operative deaths	5-Year survival rate[b] (%)
p_0	105	6	46.0*
p_1	134	7	46.0*
p_2	93	6	16.2
p_3	73	5	7.0
Total	405	24	32.2 ± 2.4

* Significant compared with p_2 and p_3 groups ($p < 0.05$).
[a] Excluding cases of low-grade malignant cancer.
[b] Excluding cases of early postoperative death.
(NCCH, Tokyo (1962–1971)).

invaded the visceral pleura, but not the parietal pleura or adjacent organs (p_2). Twelve of the 87 operative survivors in this group with p_2 disease survived more than 5 years and the relative survival rate was 16.2%. There were 73 patients (18.0%) whose tumor had infiltrated the adjacent organs such as the chest wall and mediastinum (p_3). The relative 5-year survival rate in operative survivors with p_3 disease was 7.0% (4/68).

DISCUSSION

One thousand and thirty-five patients were treated for lung cancer during the 9-year period from May, 1962 to May, 1971. Of these, 412 patients underwent pulmonary resection, and 112 patients (including 7 patients with carcinoma of low-grade malignancy) survived for 5 years or longer. The age and sex distribution of our patients did not differ greatly from those reported in the literature (5, 14).

The extent and histologic type of disease are two major factors in estimating survival. In order to clarify the extent of disease, the TNM system is now widely used throughout the world. The system, however, appears to deserve further evaluation. The number of cases assigned to Stage II was disproportionately small in our series. Since similar observations have been made by other investigators (4), it may well be a constant finding with this staging system.

Of 412 resected cases, squamous cell carcinoma represented 36.9% and adenocarcinoma 41.3%. The relative incidence of these tumors is quite close. It was previously believed that the relative incidence of adenocarcinoma is higher in Japan than in western countries. However, it has been found that the relative incidence for different cell types of lung cancer in Japan is not very different from that seen in U.S.A. This observation was made in a cooperative study between the Memorial Sloan-Kettering Cancer Center, New York, and the National Cancer Center Hospital, Tokyo. All clinical data and representative sections of lung cancers treated in these two representative cancer hospitals in the two countries were exchanged for study, reviewed, and reclassified according to the established common histological criteria. It now appears that the concept of relative predominance of adenocarcinoma in Japan has been altered (1).

The cell type of lung cancer seems to correlate with prognosis. It has been well recognized that squamous cell carcinoma shows a rather favorable survival following pulmonary resection, whereas the 5-year survival was best in patients with squamous cell carcinoma, those with small cell carcinoma did worst. All 7 patients with cancer of low-grade malignancy survived more than 5 years. The survival rates for small cell carcinoma in our series were better than those found in the literature. All of our 5-year survivors with small cell carcinoma were either in Stage I or Stage II. Their cell types were not of the "oat cell" but "others" in the WHO classification. They, on review of the sections, belonged to other groups, such as poorly differentiated squamous cell carcinoma of the small cell type, which were lumped as "intermediate cell type" in the NCCH classification. Although pulmonary resection has been considered not to be indicated for patients with small cell carcinoma, there appears to be an operative indication for a group of patients with small cell carcinoma of the intermediate cell type, which is histologically a carcinoma consisting predominantly of small cells with some features of squamous cell carcinoma, adenocarcinoma or carcinoid tumor. Paulson reported his experience with long-term survivors with small cell carcinoma. His 3 cases had to be reclassified as atypical carcinoid when he reviewed the results (12). There seems to be an obvious need for standardization concerning histological classification of subgroups of small cell carcinoma and their relation to prognosis.

It is well recognized that the presence or absence of lymph node metastasis and pleural invasion are major factors in estimating survival. The survival rates differ only slightly between the groups of patients with p_0 and p_1 disease. Survivals between those with n_0 and n_2 disease show a similar trend. p_2 or p_3, however, significantly lowered the 5-year survival rate. p_3, which indicates direct tumor invasion into the parietal pleura and adjacent organs, carried a grave prognosis. There were, however, 5 long-term survivors with p_3 disease; in all, the tumor invasion was into the chest wall. Once other adjacent vital structures such as the diaphragm, pericardium, and left atrium were involved, prognosis became very poor, and there were no long-term survivors in this situation. The 5-year survival rate in patients with n_3 disease did not exceed 10% in a majority of the reported series. Naruke (11), however, reported 13.0% (6/46) 5-year survival rate in patients with n_3 disease who underwent relatively curative resection. Bergh (2) indicated that the presence or absence of perinodal invasion has a significant influence on survival. This was not investigated in our study.

Agreement has not been reached with regard to evaluation and classification of the extent of lymph node metastasis, pleural invasion, and invasion to the neighboring structures. A map of the lymph nodes in the thorax with their station numbers was originally introduced at the NCCH in 1968 (7) (Fig. 1-A, 1-B, 1-C). In each case of lung cancer, all the dissected lymph nodes, i.e., pulmonary, interlobar, hilar, and mediastinal, have been designated with their respective station number as defined in the map.

Finally, various surgical adjuvants deserve some comment, though the data have not been presented in this report. The benefit of chemotherapy in lung cancer has not been settled. Shields (13) and Brunner (3) did not find any significant effect of chemotherapy, whereas Katsuki (8) showed beneficial effect of a long-term chemotherapy. As for immunotherapy, McNeally (10) showed intrapleural innoculation of BCG after surgery to be beneficial for Stage I disease. A randomized controlled study is being undertaken at our institution to investigate the effect of adjuvant BCG therapy, in which

S. ISHIKAWA ET AL.

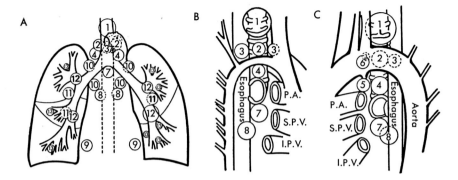

Fig. 1. A, Site of lymph nodes: 1, superior mediastinum; 2, paratracheal; 3, preretrotracheal; 4, tracheobroncheal; 5, subaortic; 6, para-aortic; 7, subcarinal; 8, paraesophageal; 9, pulmonary ligament; 10, main bronchus; 11, interlobar, 12, lobar bronchus; 13, segmental bronchus.

 B, Site of lymph nodes in the right mediastinum. P.A., pulmonary artery; S.P.V., superior pulmonary vein; I.P.V., inferior pulmonary vein.

 C, Site of lymph nodes in the left mediastinum.

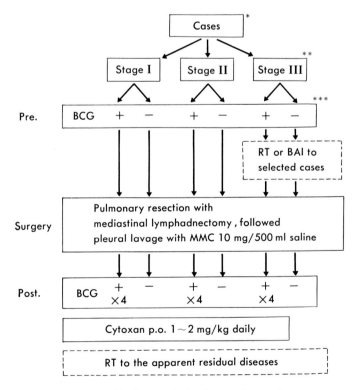

Fig. 2. Protocol-NCC-7501, for surgical adjuvant immuotherapy
 * presumed to be resectable; ** according to A.J.C.; *** randomized by envelope method. RT, radiation therapy; BAI, bronchial arterial infusion with anticancer drugs; MMC, mitomycin C.

a slightly different protocol is used for Stage I and II diseases, and for Stage III disease (Fig. 2).

Long-term survival depends as much on the correlation between host resistance and tumor growth potential as the extent of disease and histological types in surgical intervention. We believe that the tumor must be removed, if possible, and that maximum tumor reduction must be attempted even by palliative or incomplete resection. It seems equally important to extend the scope of the operative procedure or to combine surgical resection with various adjuvants such as immunotherapy, radiation, or chemotherapy in order to offer the patient every hope of long-term survival.

REFERENCES

1. Beattie, E. J., Jr. and Ishikawa, S. Memorial Sloan-Kettering Cancer Center, New Yrok and National Cancer Center, Tokyo Co-operative Lung Cancer Study. Unpublished data.
2. Bergh, N. P. and Schersten, T. Bronchogenic carcinoma. *Acta Chir. Scand.*, (*Suppl.*), **347**, 8 (1965).
3. Brunner, K. W., Marthaler, T., and Muller, W. Effect of long-term adjuvant chemotherapy with cyclophosphamide for radically resected bronchogenic carcinoma. *Cancer Chemother. Rep.* Part 3, **4**, 125–132 (1973).
4. Carr, T. D. and Mountain, C. F. The staging of lung cancer. *Sem. Oncol.*, **1**, 229–234 (1974).
5. "Description Manual for Lung Cancer Surgery," Japan Lung Cancer Society (1968).
6. Ishikawa, S. "Atlas of Lung Cancer," Nakayama Shoten, Tokyo, p. 301 (1968).
7. Ishikawa, S. "Atlas of Lung Cancer," Nakayama Shoten, Tokyo, p. 16 (1968).
8. Katsuki, H., Shimada, K., Koyama, A., Okita, M., Yamaguchi, Y., Okamoto, T., and Benfield, J. R. Long-term intermittent adjuvant chemotherapy for primary, resected lung cancer. *J. Thorac. Cardiovasc. Surg.*, **70**, 590–599 (1975).
9. Kreiberg, L., Liebow, A. A., and Uchlinger, E. A. "Histological Typing of Lung Tumors," World Health Organization, Geneva (1967).
10. McNeally, M. F., Maver, C., and Kausel, H. W. Regional immunotherapy of lung cancer with intrapleural BCG. *Lancet*, **i**, 377–379 (1976).
11. Naruke, T., Suemasu, K., and Ishikawa, S. Surgical treatment for lung cancer with metastasis to mediastinal lymph nodes. *J. Thorac. Cardiovasc. Surg.*, **71**, 279–285 (1976).
12. Paulson, D. L. and Reish, J. S. Long-term survival after resection for bronchogenic carcinoma. *Ann. Surg.*, **184**, 324 (1976).
13. Shields, T. W. Status report of adjuvant cancer chemotherapy trials in the treatment of bronchial carcinoma. *Cancer Chemother. Rep.* Part 3, **4**, 119–124 (1973).
14. Thompson, V. C. Present position relating to cancer of the lung; result of resection. *Thorax*, **15**, 5–6 (1960).
15. "TNM Classification of Malignant Tumors," 2nd Ed., International Union Against Cancer, Geneva, p. 97 (1974).

CANCER OF THE STOMACH IN JAPAN

Kiyoshi Miwa

*Department of Surgery, Gunma Prefectural Cancer Center Hospital**

Treatment results of stomach carcinoma in Japan, including the operative mortality and survival for 5 years, were studied on 5,706 patients who underwent gastrectomy during the 4 years from 1963 to 1966. These patients were registered as primary stomach carcinoma cases, confirmed histologically, and the detailed records of the individual patients, based on the General Rules for Gastric Cancer Study in Surgery and Pathology (Japanese Research Society for Gastric Cancer, 1962), were collected in the National Cancer Center, Tokyo, from 103 hospitals and computer processed. Survival was computed as the relative survival rate according to the international standard, excluding operative deaths occurring 30 days or less after gastrectomy. Among these 5,706 patients, operative deaths occurred in 231 cases and the operative mortality was 4.0%; 2,138 patients (39.1%) survived over 5 years and their relative 5-year survival rate was 44.3%. Their treatment results were analyzed relative to the sex, degree of penetration into the stomach wall by the primary tumor, lymph node metastasis, peritoneal disseminating metastasis, liver metastasis, stage of disease, type of gastrectomy, and radicality of surgery. The treatment results in the patients whose carcinoma was limited to the mucosa or submucosa, the so-called early gastric carcinoma, were so good that their relative 5-year survival rates were more than 90%. The more deeply the stomach wall was invaded, the worse became the treatment result of the patients. In contrast, operative mortality in the patients with early gastric carcinoma was fairly low (1.7 or 2.8%) but high in the patients whose carcinoma invaded neighboring organs (6.9%). In conclusion, the treatment results of stomach carcinoma in Japan have recently remarkably improved compared with the results of those treated before 1960, because of the progress and spread of the early diagnostic methods and surgical treatment.

In the past, many reports on the results of stomach carcinoma treatment have been reported by various hospitals and institutes in Japan but their data could not be compared or summed up together, because those studies were not based on unified rules for grading the extent of the disease, classifying the type of carcinoma, describing the treatment method, or calculating the treatment result. To overcome this situation, the Japanese Research Society for Gastric Cancer was organized and General Rules for Gastric Cancer Study in Surgery and Pathology was published by this Society in 1962 (*1, 4, 5*) (hereinafter abbreviated as the General Rules). Since then, these rules have rapidly spread and have been widely used in Japan.

* Takabayashi 617-1, Oota 373, Gunma, Japan (三輪 潔).

TABLE I. Treatment Results of 5,706 Patinets

	No. of patients	Operative death within 30 days		No. of patients excluding operat. death	1	
		No. of cases	Op.M. (%)		No. of cases	R.S.R. (%)
Males	3,771	179	4.7	3,592	2,499	71.4
Females	1,935	52	2.7	1,883	1,351	73.3
Total	5,706	231	4.0	5,475	3,850	71.9

Op.M., operative mortality; R.S.R., relative survival rate.

Registration of patients with stomach cancer was planned by this Society in 1968 and the registration form was established to fill in detailed data according to the General Rules, including follow-up data for individual patients. The registration started, simultaneously, retrospectively for the patients treated in 1963 and prospectively for the patients treated in 1969, and the registration is still under way for new patients with stomach cancer.

The completed registration cards from all over the country have been collected in the National Cancer Center, Tokyo, and detailed records of individual patients have been computer processed (HITAC 8350, Hitachi, Ltd., Tokyo). The treatment results, including operative mortality, were calculated and analyzed by the computer. Survival was computed as the relative survival rate in accordance with the international standard (2, 3), excluding operative deaths occurring 30 days or less after surgical operation.

During 4 years from 1963 to 1966, there were 6,050 cases whose stomach carcinoma was resected surgically among 8,411 patients registered from 103 hospitals as primary cases of stomach carcinoma confirmed histologically, and their resectability was 71.9%. Among these, 235 patients who had double cancers in the stomach or other organs were excluded from this series for lack of sufficient information concerning other cancers on the registration form. Consequently, 5,815 cases were used in this study, but 109 of these cases were further excluded by computer analysis as being unsuitable for calculating the relative survival rate, because the date of birth or surgery was incomplete. Finally, 5,706 resected cases were studied for the results of recent treatment of stomach carcinoma in Japan.

Sex

The relative survival rate of all patients undergoing gastrectomy, excluding 231 operative deaths (4.0%), was 71.9% at 12 months, 56.0% at 24 months, 49.5% at 36 months, 46.4% at 48 months, and 44.3% at 60 months. Although 48 of these cases were lost to follow-up within 5 postoperative years, they were calculated as a half survivor according to the international rule, since they were no more than 1% of the entire series. Among the 5,706 patients, 3,771 cases (or 66.1%) were males and 1,935 cases (or 33.9%) were females. Operative deaths of males occurred in 179 patients (4.7%) and 52 deaths (2.7%) in females. The relative 5-year survival rate was 44.6% in males and 43.6% in females, there being no statistical difference between the sexes (Table I).

with Stomach Carcinoma by Sex

Survival after gastrectomy (years)							
2		3		4		5	
No. of cases	R.S.R. (%)	No. of cases	R.S.R. (%)	No. of cases	R.S.R. (%)	No. of cases	R.S.R. (%)
1,908	56.0	1,660	50.1	1,498	46.6	1,377	44.6
1,022	55.9	891	49.3	815	45.8	761	43.6
2,930	56.0	2,551	49.5	2,313	46.4	2,138	44.3

Penetration and Extent of the Primary Tumor

In accordance with the General Rules, the degree of penetration into the stomach wall by the primary tumor is divided into the following categories: Mucosa (m), subserosa (sm), tunica muscularis propriae (pm), subserosa (ss), and serosa; the degree of invasion into the stomach serosa is subdivided into the three categories of s_1, s_2, and s_3. The sign s_1 is used for infiltration extending into the serosa but confined to the serosa and covered by a connective tissue, s_2 for carcinoma tissue lying adjacent to the serosa or exposed on the surface of the serosa, and s_3 for carcinoma crossing over the serosa and extending to neighboring organs.

The patients with carcinoma confined to the mucosa had a relative survival rate of 101.6% at 5 years which means that mortality in this group is almost the same as the normal mortality rate of the corresponding age group. The relative 5-year survival rates of the patients with the tumor involving submucosa, muscularis propriae, and subserosa were respectively 90.3%, 70.2%, and 49.8%. In the patients

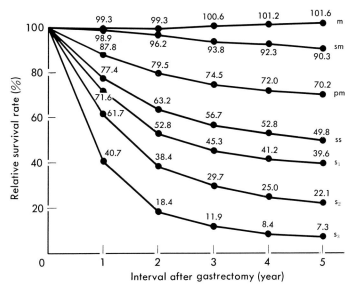

Fig. 1. Survival curve of patients with stomach carcinoma according to stomach wall penetration and serosal invasion by the primary tumor

TABLE II. Treatment Results of 5,706 Patients with Stomach Carcinoma According

	No. of patients	Operative death within 30 days		No. of potients excluding operat. death	1	
		No. of cases	Op.M. (%)		No. of cases	R.S.P. (%)
Mucosa (m)	362	6	1.7	356	346	99.3
Submucosa (sm)	433	12	2.8	421	409	98.9
Muscularis prop. (pm)	658	26	4.0	632	544	87.8
Subserosa (ss)	796	30	3.8	766	580	77.4
Serosa 1 (s_1)	752	27	3.6	725	506	71.6
Serosa 2 (s_2)	1,515	59	3.9	1,456	881	61.7
Serosa 3 (s_3)	565	39	6.9	526	210	40.7
Unknown	625	32	5.1	593	374	(63.1)
Total	5,706	231	4.0	5,475	3,850	71.9

Figures in parentheses are crude survival rate assuming the cases lost to follow-up as dead.

with tumor invading the serosa, the relative 5-year survival rate was 39.6% for the s_1 group, 22.1% for the s_2 group, and 7.3% for the s_3 group (Table II). The treatment results in patients whose carcinoma is limited to the mucosa or mucosa and submucosa, the so-called early gastric carcinoma, is extremely good, but the more deeply the stomach wall is invaded, the worse becomes the treatment result of the patients. In contrast, operative mortality in patients with early gastric carcinoma (m, sm) is fairly low (1.7% or 2.8%) but is high in the case of s_3 (6.9%), in which it was necessary to carry out combined resection of the neighboring organs to complete radical surgery for cancer. The survival curves are shown in Fig. 1 and the curves correspond respectively from higher to lower to m, sm, pm, ss, s_1, s_2, and s_3.

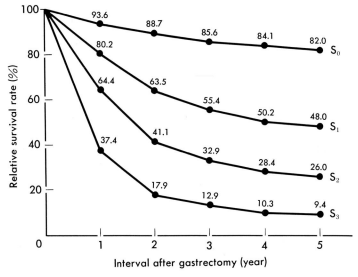

FIG. 2. Survival curve of patients with stomach carcinoma according to macroscopic serosal involvement by the primary tumor

to Stomach Wall Penetration and Serosal Invasion by the Primary Tumor

Survival after gastrectomy (years)							
2		3		4		5	
No. of cases	R.S.R. (%)	No. of cases	R.S.R. (%)	No. of cases	R.S.R. (%)	No. of cases	R.S.R. (%)
339	99.3	337	100.6	331	101.2	324	101.6
389	96.2	371	93.8	357	92.3	340	90.3
481	79.5	440	74.5	414	72.0	390	70.2
463	63.2	407	56.7	370	52.8	335	49.8
364	52.8	305	45.3	270	41.2	250	39.6
538	38.4	408	29.7	338	25.0	292	22.1
93	18.4	59	11.9	40	8.4	34	7.3
263	(44.4)	224	(37.8)	193	(32.5)	173	(29.2)
2,930	56.0	2,551	49.5	2,313	46.4	2,138	44.3

The degree of invasion of the primary tumor into the serosa is also macroscopically divided into 4 groups in the same manner and these are expressed as S_0, S_1, S_2, and S_3. S_1 means that the invasion into the serosa is macroscopically suspected and S_2 means that the serosal invasion is macroscopically defined. The relative 5-year survival rate was 82.0%, 48.0%, 26.0%, and 9.4%, respectively, for the group of S_0, S_1, S_2, and S_3 (Fig. 2).

Lymph Node Metastasis

According to the General Rules, regional lymph nodes are divided, in principle, into 4 groups as follows: Group 1 includes strictly perigastric lymph nodes including right and left cardiac, lesser, and greater curvature, and supra- and infra-pyloric nodes; Group 2 is more distant than Group 1 and includes the lymph nodes located along the left gastric, common hepatic and splenic arteries as well as around the celiac artery and splenic hilus; Group 3 is more distant than Group 2 and includes the lymph nodes located in hepatoduodenal ligament, on the posterior aspect of the pancreas, at the root of mesenterium, and at the diaphragm and paraesophageal nodes on lower part of thorax; and Group 4 includes all lymph nodes located further away than Group 3. These principles are applicable only when the tumor occupies a major part of the stomach and, when the tumor is localized in the minor part of the stomach, several modifications taking into consideration the stream of lymph are made according to the General Rules. If a major part of the primary tumor is localized in the upper third portion of the stomach, including the cardiac area and fundus, supra- and infra-pyloric lymph nodes must be changed to Group 2 from Group 1. When the tumor is mostly localized in the middle third of the stomach, the left cardiac lymph node is changed to Group 2 from Group 1, and the diaphragmatic and paraesophageal nodes to Group 4 from Group 3. When the tumor is mostly localized in the lower third of the stomach, including the antral area, the right cardiac node is changed to Group 2 from Group 1, the left cardiac node to Group 3 from Group 1, the nodes at the splenic hilus and

TABLE III.   Treatment Results of 5,706 Patients with Stomach Carcinoma

	No. of patients	Operative death within 30 days		No. of patients excluding operat. death	1	
		No. of cases	Op.M. (%)		No. of cases	R.S.R. (%)
n (−)	1,592	58	3.6	1,534	1,404	93.6
n$_1$ (+)	1,404	46	3.3	1,358	944	71.0
n$_2$ (+)	1,119	51	4.6	1,068	620	59.4
n$_3$ (+)	260	11	4.2	249	112	46.1
n$_4$ (+)	71	5	7.0	66	20	30.8
Unknown	1,260	60	4.8	1,200	750	(62.5)
Total	5,706	231	4.0	5,475	3,850	71.9

Figures in parentheses are crude survival rate assuming the cases lost to follow-up as dead.

along the splenic artery to Group 3 from Group 2, and the diaphragmatic and para-esophageal nodes to Group 4 from Group 3.

The relative 5-year survival rate of the patients with no metastasis to the lymph node (n(−)) was 79.5% and that of the patients with metastasis to the lymph nodes of Group 1 (n$_1$(+)) was 38.5%, that of Group 2 (n$_2$(+)) was 22.8%, that of Group 3 (n$_3$(+)) was 11.1%, and that of Group 4 (n$_4$(+)) was 8.5% (Table III). These metastases were confirmed by histological examination of lymph nodes removed at the time of operation.

On the other hand, when the metastasis to lymph nodes is graded according to the macroscopic, prior to microscopic findings, the grade is expressed as N(−), N$_1$(+), N$_2$(+), N$_3$(+), and N$_4$(+). In this series, the relative 5-year survival rate of these

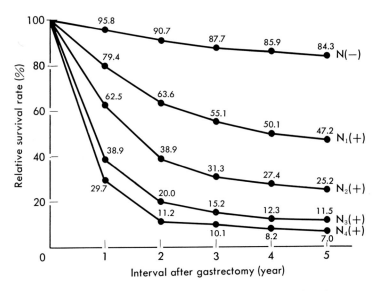

FIG. 3.   Survival curve of patients with stomach carcinoma according to macro-scopic lymph node metastases

According to Lymph Node Metastases Confirmed Histologically

Survival after gastrectomy (years)							
2		3		4		5	
No. of cases	R.S.R. (%)	No. of cases	R.S.R. (%)	No. of cases	R.S.R. (%)	No. of cases	R.S.R. (%)
1,285	87.4	1,217	84.5	1,151	81.8	1,084	79.5
683	52.5	572	45.0	502	40.4	465	38.5
371	36.2	277	27.8	239	24.6	214	22.8
57	23.9	38	16.2	33	14.4	25	11.1
9	14.1	7	11.2	6	9.9	5	8.5
525	(43.8)	440	(36.7)	382	(31.8)	345	(28.8)
2,930	56.0	2,551	49.5	2,313	46.4	2,138	44.3

patients was 84.3% for $N(-)$, 47.2% for $N_1(+)$, 25.2% for $N_2(+)$, 11.5% for $N_3(+)$, and 7.0% for $N_4(+)$. The survival curves according to the macroscopic grading are shown in Fig. 3. This grading is less accurate than the histological grading but will be usable for any surgeon and at any hospital in which histological examination of lymph nodes is impossible.

Disseminating Metastasis to the Peritoneum

The degree of the disseminating metastasis to the peritoneum is divided into four categories according to the General Rules. P_1 shows that disseminating metastasis is found macroscopically at the adjacent peritoneum which is above the transverse colon, including the gastrocolic omentum but excluding the abdominal surface of the diaphragm, P_2 shows few metastases are found at the distant peritoneum below the transverse colon and the abdominal surface of the diaphragm, and P_3 shows numerous metastases to the adjacent and distant peritoneum. P_0 means that there is no disseminating metastasis to any serosal surface.

The relative 5-year survival rate of the patients with P_1 was 12.4%. Among 293 patients with P_2, there were 14 patients surviving over 5 years after gastrectomy and their relative 5-year survival rate was 5.3%. None of 120 patients with P_3 survived over 4 years in spite of palliative gastrectomy. On the other hand, the relative 5-year survival rate of the patients with no disseminating metastasis to the peritoneum (P_0) was 53.5% (Table IV).

Disseminating metastasis to the peritoneum is one of the important factors which make the patients' prognosis worse but there are some possibilities for curing patients with P_1 by combined complete removal of the gastrocolic and gastrohepatic omentum and the peritoneum of the bursa omentalis. Moreover, when few disseminations are found at the retrovesical or retrouterine pouch (P_2) but no unremovable metastasis to a lymph node and no liver metastasis is found, gastrectomy should be carried out, since macroscopic judgement for disseminating metastasis is not always correct.

TABLE IV. Treatment Results of 5,706 Patients with Stomach

| | No. of patients | Operative death within 30 days | | No. of patients excluding operat. death | 1 | |
		No. of cases	Op.M. (%)		No. of cases	R.S.R. (%)
P_0	4,480	155	3.5	4,325	3,377	79.9
P_1	697	45	6.5	652	309	48.5
P_2	315	22	7.0	293	99	34.6
P_3	124	4	3.2	120	16	13.8
Unknown	90	5	5.6	85	49	(57.6)
Total	5,706	231	4.0	5,475	3,850	71.9

Figures in parentheses are crude survival rate assuming the cases lost to follow-up as dead.

TABLE V. Treatment Results of 5,706 Patients with Stomach

| | No. of patients | Operative death within 30 days | | No. of patients excluding operat. death | 1 | |
		No. of cases	Op.M. (%)		No. of cases	R.S.R. (%)
H_0	5,369	205	3.8	5,164	3,757	74.4
H_1	144	12	8.3	132	47	36.4
H_2	93	8	8.6	85	11	13.4
H_3	48	3	6.3	45	4	9.3
Unknown	52	3	5.8	49	31	(63.3)
Total	5,706	231	4.0	5,475	3,850	71.9

Figures in parentheses are crude survival rate assuming the cases lost to follow-up as dead.

Metastasis to the Liver

According to the General Rules, the degree of metastasis to the liver is divided into 4 groups as follows: H_0 shows no liver metastasis; H_1 shows metastasis limited to one of the liver lobes; H_2 a few metastases to both lobes; and H_3 numerous scattered metastases to both lobes.

Ten of 132 patients with liver metastasis graded as H_1 and one of 85 patients with H_2 survived more than 5 years after gastrectomy, with or without removal of a liver metastasis. Although some may not have been judged correctly for liver metastasis because of macroscopic judgement, metastasis to the liver was confirmed histologically in one case of H_1 removed by partial hepatectomy and he survived over 5 years without recurrence of cancer. Another patient with liver metastasis of H_1, not removed surgically but that had been slowly growing after palliative gastrectomy, survived for 5 years and died 3 months later of cachexia of cancer. With the exception of these patients, metastasis to the liver is the most important factor which causes the patients' prognosis to become worse. In the present series, 90% of the 144 patients with H_1 died within 30 months in spite of gastrectomy, with 12 operative deaths, 90% of the 93 patients with H_2 died within 15 months including 8 operative deaths, and 90% of the 48 patients with H_3 died within 12 months including 3 operative deaths (Table

Carcinoma According to Peritoneal Disseminating Metastasis

Survival after gastrectomy (years)							
2		3		4		5	
No. of cases	R.S.R. (%)	No. of cases	R.S.R. (%)	No. of cases	R.S.R. (%)	No. of cases	R.S.R. (%)
2,701	65.3	2,388	59.1	2,188	55.5	2,038	53.5
155	24.8	117	19.2	89	14.9	72	12.4
36	12.8	21	7.6	18	6.6	14	5.3
4	3.6	1	0.9	0	—	—	—
34	(40.0)	24	(28.2)	18	(21.2)	14	(16.5)
2,930	56.0	2,551	49.5	2,313	46.4	2,138	44.3

Carcinoma According to Liver Metastasis

Survival after gastrectomy (years)							
2		3		4		5	
No. of cases	R.S.R. (%)	No. of cases	R.S.R. (%)	No. of cases	R.S.R. (%)	No. of cases	R.S.R. (%)
2,889	58.5	2,520	52.2	2,289	48.6	2,116	46.5
18	14.3	13	10.6	11	9.3	10	8.7
3	3.8	2	2.6	1	1.3	1	1.3
0	—	—	—	—	—	—	—
20	(40.8)	16	(32.7)	12	(24.5)	11	(22.4)
2,930	56.0	2,551	49.5	2,313	46.4	2,183	44.3

V). In contrast, the relative survival rate of 5,164 patients without macroscopic metastasis to the liver was 46.5% at 60 months.

Stage of Stomach Cancer

The stage of stomach cancer is expressed by the General Rules from the corresponding stages of the peritoneal metastasis, liver metastasis, lymph node metastasis, and serosal invasion, obtained separately in accordance with Table VI, and the highest among them becomes the representative stage. Although degrees of peritoneal disseminating metastasis and liver metastasis are always based on macroscopic findings, in the

TABLE VI. Histological Staging Based on the General Rules in Japan

Stage	Peritoneal disseminating metastasis	Liver metastasis	Lymph node metastasis	Serosal invasion
I	P_0	H_0	n (−)	s_0
II	P_0	H_0	n_1 (+), n_2 (+)	s_1
III	P_0	H_0	n_3 (+)	s_2
IV	More than P_1	More than H_1	n_4 (+)	s_3

TABLE VII.   Treatment Results of 5,706 Patients with

	No. of patients	Operative death within 30 days		No. of patients excluding operat. death	1	
		No. of cases	Op.M. (%)		No. of cases	R.S.R. (%)
I	1,043	27	2.6	1,016	981	98.6
II	1,104	34	3.1	1,070	886	84.7
III	939	29	3.1	910	634	71.1
IV	1,629	106	6.5	1,523	617	41.5
Unknown	991	35	3.5	956	732	(76.6)
Total	5,706	231	4.0	5,475	3,850	71.9

Figures in parentheses are crude survival rate assuming the cases lost to follow-up as dead.

case of histological staging, grades of lymph node metastasis and serosal invasion are based on microscopic findings, but macroscopic staging is based on macroscopic findings.

Among 5,706 patients given gastrectomy, 1,043 patients (18.3%) belonged to histological Stage I, 1,104 (19.3%) to Stage II, 939 (16.5%) to Stage III, and 1,629 (28.5%) to Stage IV. Histological staging for the remaining 991 patients was undetermined due to lack of histological examination. The relative 5-year survival rate was 94.4% for Stage I, 56.1% for Stage II, 30.1% for Stage III, and 9.3% for Stage IV (Table VII).

In the case of macroscopic staging, the relative 5-year survival rate was 95.3% in 953 patients with Stage I, 62.0% in 1,418 patients in Stage II, 33.2% in 1,417 patients in Stage III and 10.4% in 1,773 patients in Stage IV. Their survival curves are shown in Fig. 4.

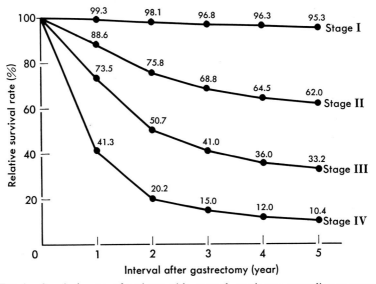

FIG. 4.   Survival curve of patients with stomach carcinoma according to macroscopic stage

Stomach Carcinoma According to Histological Stage

| Survival after gastrectomy (years) | | | | | | | |
| 2 | | 3 | | 4 | | 5 | |
No. of cases	R.S.R. (%)	No. of cases	R.S.R. (%)	No. of cases	R.S.R. (%)	No. of cases	R.S.R. (%)
946	97.0	917	96.2	888	95.2	852	94.4
718	70.2	627	62.8	567	58.4	527	56.1
423	48.3	331	38.6	281	33.4	248	30.1
289	19.9	204	14.3	154	11.1	127	9.3
554	(57.9)	470	(49.2)	423	(44.2)	384	(40.2)
2,930	56.0	2,551	49.5	2,313	46.4	2,138	44.3

Type of Gastrectomy

According to the extent of the resected stomach, gastrectomy is classified by the General Rules into total, proximal subtotal, proximal regular, distal subtotal, and distal regular gastrectomy. Subtotal gastrectomy means the removal of 4/5 or more of the stomach and regular gastrectomy means the removal of less than 4/5 of the stomach.

Among the 5,706 resected cases, total gastrectomy was carried out in 933 patients (16.4%) and their relative 5-year survival rate was 19.8%, excluding 58 operative deaths (6.2%). Proximal gastrectomy was carried out in 327 patients (5.7%), in which proximal subtotal gastrectomy was carried out in 122 patients (2.1%) and their relative 5-year survival rate was 41.5%, excluding 9 operative deaths (7.4%), and proximal regular gastrectomy was carried out in 205 patients (7.6%) and their relative 5-year survival rate was 26.5%, excluding 21 operative deaths (10.2%). Among the 4,322 patients undergoing distal gastrectomy (75.7%), distal subtotal gastrectomy was carried out in 1,690 patients (28.2%) and their relative 5-year survival rate was 45.8%, excluding 50 operative deaths (3.1%), and distal regular gastrectomy was carried out in 2,713 patients (47.6%) and their relative 5-year survival rate was 52.9%, excluding 85 operative deaths (3.1%). Atypical gastrectomy including segmental gastrectomy and surgical polypectomy was carried out in 38 patients and they had a relative 5-year survival rate of 72.1% (Table VIII). Since the extent of gastrectomy is related to the extent of disease, it is impossible to evaluate the type of gastrectomy for treatment method by these end results but operative death is more frequent in total and proximal gastrectomy than distal gastrectomy.

Radicality of Surgical Treatment

According to the General Rules, radicality of the surgical resection of stomach cancer is classified into two categories of "curative resection" and "noncurative resection." These are subdivided into two groups; "absolute" curative resection means that there is no metastasis to the peritoneum or the liver and no cancer infiltration at the margins of surgical excision of the stomach; the degree of serosal invasion is s_2 or less, or a suitable combined resection of the neighboring organ is carried out when the

TABLE VIII. Treatment Results of 5,706 Patients with

	No. of patients	Operative death within 30 days		No. of patients excluding operat. death	1	
		No. of cases	Op.M. (%)		No. of cases	R.S.R. (%)
Total	933	58	6.2	875	463	54.1
Proximal	327	30	9.2	297	178	61.3
Subtotal	122	9	7.4	113	69	62.3
Regular	205	21	10.2	184	109	60.7
Distal	4,322	135	3.1	4,187	3,142	76.7
Subtotal	1,609	50	3.1	1,559	1,133	74.4
Regular	2,713	85	3.1	2,628	2,009	78.0
Atypical	38	0	—	38	29	77.5
Unknown	86	8	9.3	78	38	(48.7)
Total	5,706	231	4.0	5,475	3,850	71.9

Figures in parentheses are crude survival rate assuming the cases lost to follow-up as dead.

TABLE IX. Treatment Results of 5,706 Patients with Stomach

	No. of patients	Operative death within 30 days		No. of patients excluding operat. death	1	
		No. of cases	Op.M. (%)		No. of cases	R.S.R. (%)
Curative resection	3,056	93	3.0	2,963	2,545	87.8
Absolute	2,010	62	3.1	1,948	1,784	93.6
Relative	1,046	31	3.0	1,015	761	76.5
Noncurat. resection	1,739	98	5.6	1,641	691	43.0
Relative	475	19	4.0	456	275	61.7
Absolute	1,264	79	6.3	1,185	416	35.8
Unknown	911	40	4.4	871	614	(70.5)
Total	5,706	231	4.0	5,475	3,850	71.9

Figures in parentheses are crude survival rate assuming the cases lost to follow-up as dead.

serosal invasion is s_3, and dissection is made for the more distant group of lymph nodes than the group with confirmed metastasis, or dissection is made of the group of n_1 or more when there is no metastasis to the lymph nodes. If the number of the group of lymph nodes dissected is equal to the number of the group with a metastasis, such a curative gastrectomy is classified as "relative" curative resection. The case beyond the definition of both curative resections is called noncurative resection, in which the case with a possible complete removal of cancer is classified as relative noncurative resection and, if cancer cells clearly remain, the case is classified as absolute noncurative resection.

In relation to the above-mentioned conditions, when macroscopic findings are used instead of microscopic findings concerning lymph node metastasis, serosal involvement and infiltration to the margins of surgical excision, the terms "macroscopically" absolute or relative curative resection and "macroscopically" relative or absolute noncurative resection are used in the General Rules.

Stomach Carcinoma According the Type of Gastrectomy

Survival after gastrectomy (years)							
2		3		4		5	
No. of cases	R.S.R. (%)	No. of cases	R.S.R. (%)	No. of cases	R.S.R. (%)	No. of cases	R.S.R. (%)
281	33.3	214	25.8	176	21.7	158	19.8
127	44.9	107	38.9	94	35.2	80	32.1
54	50.5	47	45.7	43	43.7	37	41.5
73	41.4	60	34.7	51	30.1	43	26.5
2,469	61.6	2,180	55.7	1,996	52.3	1,857	50.3
872	58.4	762	52.3	686	48.3	633	45.8
1,597	63.6	1,418	57.7	1,310	54.7	1,224	52.9
26	70.5	25	69.1	25	70.5	24	72.1
27	(34.6)	25	(32.1)	22	(28.2)	19	(24.4)
2,930	56.0	2,551	49.5	2,313	46.4	2,138	44.3

Carcinoma According to the Microscopic Radicality of Surgical Treatment

Survival after gastrectomy (years)							
2		3		4		5	
No. of cases	R.S.R. (%)	No. of cases	R.S.R. (%)	No. of cases	R.S.R. (%)	No. of cases	R.S.R. (%)
2,160	76.1	1,945	70.0	1,799	66.3	1,692	64.2
1,615	86.6	1,500	82.2	1,407	78.9	1,331	77.0
545	56.0	445	46.7	392	42.0	361	39.8
329	20.9	225	14.7	184	12.3	149	10.4
154	35.4	117	27.5	106	25.6	88	22.3
175	15.4	108	9.7	78	7.2	61	5.9
441	(50.6)	381	(43.7)	330	(37.9)	297	(34.1)
2,930	56.0	2,551	49.5	2,313	46.4	2,138	44.3

Among the entire 5,706 patients who underwent gastrectomy in the present series, curative resection was carried out in 3,056 patients (53.6%) and their relative 5-year survival rate was 64.2%, excluding the 93 operative deaths. On the other hand, non-curative resection was carried out in 1,739 patients (30.5%) and their relative 5-year survival rate was 10.4%, excluding the 98 operative deaths. Radicality of surgical procedure in the remaining 911 patients could not be determined owing to the lack of essential histological examination. Among the 2,010 patients who received absolute curative resection (35.2%), 1,046 patients received relative curative resection (18.3%), 475 patients received relative noncurative resection (8.3%), and 1,264 patients received absolute noncurative resection (22.2%); 62 (3.1%), 31 (3.0%), 19 (4.0%), and 79 (6.3%) deaths occurred, respectively, within 30 days after the operation, and their respective relative 5-year survival rates were 77.0%, 39.8%, 22.3%, and 5.9%, excluding operative deaths (Table IX).

On the other hand, when the radicality of surgical procedure was classified by

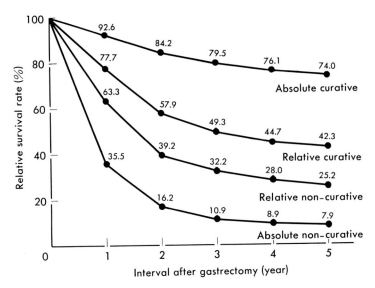

F<small>IG</small>. 5.   Survival curve of patients with stomach carcinoma according to macroscopic radicality of surgical treatment

the macroscopic instead of microscopic findings, according to the General Rules, the
relative 5-year survival rate in the case of absolute curative resection, relative curative
resection, relative noncurative resection, and absolute noncurative resection was, respectively, 74.0%, 42.3%, 25.2%, and 7.9%. The survival curves in these cases are
shown in Fig. 5.

In either microscopic or macroscopic classification, operative deaths occurred most
frequently and survival was poorest in the group of absolute noncurative resection,
which might be carried out in some expectation of chemotherapeutic effect. In contrast, operative deaths occurred less frequently and the survival was satisfactorily
greater in the group of absolute curative resection, in which the major part of early
gastric carcinoma was included.

DISCUSSION

Curability of stomach cancer by a surgical procedure depends on the relation
between the degree of advancement of cancer and surgical treatment for cancer. Therefore, the earlier the disease is diagnosed, the more completely the surgical treatment
can be carried out with a chance of cure. Contrarily, the later the disease is discovered,
the more incomplete will be the surgical treatment. However, if stomach cancer shows
a similar stage in different patients, the treatment results will be influenced by the
surgical procedure for sufficient resection of the stomach, wide dissection of the lymph
nodes, or suitable combined resection of the neighboring organs. It is necessary and
important to analyze treatment results in detail according to the relationship between
the advancement of stomach cancer including the primary tumor, metastasis, staging
etc., and the result of surgery; of special importance is the analysis of the relation between the degree of metastasis to lymph nodes and the degree of dissection of the
lymph nodes. The reason is that the dissection of lymph node metastasis in cases with

TABLE X. End Results of Stomach Carcinoma and Frequency
of Early Gastric Carcinoma in Japan

	Crude 5-year survival rate (%)		Frequency of early gastric carcinoma out of resected cases (%)
	Resected cases	Radically operated cases	
1926–1935	10±5	20±5	1
1936–1945	15±5	25±5	1
1946–1955	20±5	30±5	2
1956–1962	25±5	40±5	3–5
1963–1966[a]	39	54	10
1967–1973[a]	?	?	18

[a] Based on this registration study. Others based on previously reported literature.

a completely resectable primary tumor and without peritoneal and liver metastases is the most important procedure which a surgeon can carry out to cure the patient with stomach carcinoma. Another reason is that the accurate grasp of the relationship of these factors and the standardization of the surgical treatment based on these analyses is obligatory for evaluating the effect of various kinds of adjuvant chemotherapy. In the present series of investigation, the result of these analyses was not shown, as the registration of the patients with stomach cancer is still underway in Japan and their data based on the standardized General Rules are being stored for future publication on the results of detailed investigations.

The result of recent treatment of stomach carcinoma in Japan became clear from the present study. As compared with the past treatment results, in Japanese literature (Table X), a remarkable improvement has been made on the end result of surgical treatment for stomach cancer. Owing to the progress and spread of early diagnostic methods and adequate surgical procedures, treatment results of stomach cancer will be improved further in Japan.

Acknowledgment

This work was supported in part by a Grant-in-Aid for Cancer Research from the Ministry of Health and Welfare, Japanese Government.

REFERENCES

1. Committee on Histological Classification of Gastric Carcinoma, Japanese Society of Pathology, and Japanese Research Society for Gastric Cancer. Histological classification of gastric carcinoma. *Gann*, **61**, 93–104 (1970).
2. Cutler, S. J. Computation of survival rate. *Natl. Cancer Inst. Monogr.*, **15**, 381–385 (1964).
3. Ederer, F., Axtell, L. M., and Cutler, S. J. The relative survival rate: A statistical methodology. *Natl. Cancer Inst. Monogr.*, **6**, 101–121 (1961).
4. Japanese Research Society for Gastric Cancer. "General Rules for the Gastric Cancer Study in Surgery and Pathology," Kanehara Shuppan, Tokyo (1962) (in Japanese).
5. Japanese Research Society for Gastric Cancer. The general rules for the gastric cancer study in surgery. *Japan. J. Surg.*, **3**, 61–71 (1973).

CANCER OF THE STOMACH AT CANCER INSTITUTE HOSPITAL, TOKYO

Tamaki Kajitani and Kunio Takagi

*Department of Surgery, Cancer Institute Hospital**

Investigations were made of therapeutic results of gastric cancer operations in the Department of Surgery, Cancer Institute Hospital, Tokyo, during the 25 years from 1946 to 1970. The rate of curative operation for gastric cancer improved in the 1960's, and the 5-year survival rate also showed a marked improvement to 59%, compared to that of 40% in the 1950's. The primary factor for this improvement is the improved detection of early cancer due to the progress in stomach diagnostics. The incidence of early gastric cancer among the curative operations was about 5% in the 1950's but this incidence was over 20% in the 1960's, with a 5-year survival rate of early gastric cancer cases reaching 90%. This fact indicates the importance of early diagnosis of gastric cancer for the improvement of therapeutic results in cancer. Even in advanced cases with infiltration of cancer into the proper muscle of the gastric wall and into the serosa, selection of radical operation and/or surgical technique, especially the combined resection of the surrounding organ(s) accompanied by extended dissection of lymph nodes, has resulted in a 5-year survival rate of 42%. Cases given total gastrectomy has increased from the 1950's, with extensive dissection of lymph nodes, but death directly due to such a radical operation has been low, 3.7%, indicating that surgical treatment of gastric cancer is no longer a danger.

The incidence of gastric cancer is the highest among malignant tumors in Japan, and the corrected death rate for gastric cancer, according to Segi's statistics (*12*), was 68 for males and 35 for females per 100,000 population, in 1965. Since the end of World War II, treatment of pulmonary tuberculosis has been successful and, with the marked decrease in pulmonary tuberculosis, public concern centered on cancer, especially gastric cancer. Tremendous efforts have been made for the early detection of gastric cancer, especially in the 1960's, and progress in the double-contrast method (*13*) for X-ray examination, and introduction of a gastrocamera (*11*), fiberscope, and gastric biopsy (*14*) in endoscopy have entirely changed the mode of diagnosis of gastric cancer. In the field of surgery, extension of radical surgery, accompanying progress in surgical techniques from the 1950's, has gradually improved the surgical results of gastric cancer (*3, 8, 9*).

The present paper reviews the results of treatment of gastric cancer after World War II, centered on the results of gastric cancer patients treated in the Cancer Institute Hospital, Tokyo, during the 10 years from 1960 to 1970. From such a result, the factor

* Kami-Ikebukuro 1-37-1, Toshima-ku, Tokyo 170, Japan (梶谷 鐶, 高木国夫).

or factors contributing to the improvement of therapeutic results will be examined in order to contribute to the progress in the treatment of gastric cancer.

Number of Gastric Cancer Cases

The number of primary cases of gastric cancer hospitalized in this surgical department during the 25 years from September, 1946, when the hospital surgical department was reopened after the end of war, to December, 1970, totalled 5,104 cases, 4,988 cases of which received laparotomy. Curative operation was carried out on 3,437 cases, which constitute 67% of all hospitalized cases and 69% of laparotomied cases. Table I shows changes in the rate of curative operation on laparotomied cases during the 25 years, divided into 5-year periods. It will be seen that the rate of curative operation was low during the latter part of the 1940's but increased gradually to 77% from 1966 to 1970, with a sudden increase after 1961. This increase in the rate of curative operation is primarily due to the progress made in the diagnostic technique for gastric cancer since 1961, and to the early diagnosis of gastric cancer made possible by mass survey. As shown in Table II, this period coincides with a sudden increase in the incidence of early gastric cancer among the cases operated on.

Among 4,988 cases of laparotomy, curative operation was carried out in 3,437 cases, 92 cases (3%) of which died within 30 days after surgery, and 1,702 cases who lived for 5 years or more, the 5-year survival rate being 50%. The 5-year survival rate of solitary cancer cases was 49% (1,541/3,145) and that of multiple cancer cases was 53% (154/292).

TABLE I. Number of Cases Given Curative Operation
(1946–1970, Including Multiple Cancer)

Period	Curative operation No. of cases	Palliative operation No. of cases	Percentage of curative op. to total op. (%)
1946–1950	209	172	55 (209/381)
1951–1955	599	333	64 (599/932)
1956–1960	884	429	67 (884/1,373)
1961–1965	836 .	345	71 (836/1,181)
1966–1970	909	272	77 (909/1,181)
Total	3,437	1,551	69 (3,437/4,988)

TABLE II. Incidence of Early Gastric Cancer among Laparotomied Gastric Cancer Cases
(1946–1970, Including Multiple Cancer)

Period	Laparotomy No. of cases	Early cancer	
		No. of cases	%
1946–1950	381	5	1.0
1951–1955	932	24	2.6
1956–1960	1,313	73	5.6
1961–1965	1,181	168	14.2
1966–1970	1,181	285	24.1
Total	4,988	554	11.1

Factor(s) affecting the therapeutic result of gastric cancer will be examined in 3,144 cases of solitary cancer, excluding cases with multiple cancer.

Long-term Results of Single Gastric Cancer Cases

As shown in Table III, periodic variation in 5-year survival rate of curative operation cases was around 40% from 1946 to 1960, but increased to 55–59% from 1961. When early cancer and advanced cancer are considered separately, the 5-year survival rate in early cancer remained constant at 90%, there being no periodic change. In the case of advanced cancer, improvement in the 5-year survival rate was very small and was around 45%, even after 1961. In other words, the improvement in the therapeutic result of gastric cancer as a whole after 1966 is largely due to the increase in the number of early cancers and this fact indicates the great importance of early detection of gastric cancer in improving the end results.

Curative operation for gastric cancer has become safe owing to the progress in anesthetic and surgical techniques, as well as by the progress in medicine in general. In advanced cases, we make a wide resection 5–6 cm from the macroscopic border of gastric cancer, and total gastrectomy is carried out in the cases (26%) in which the distance from the macroscopic border of gastric cancer to the surgical stump seems insufficient. For the dissection of lymph nodes, an extended dissection as far as Group 3 (cf. Miwa's article, lymph node metastasis) is carried out. Combined resection of adjacent and surrounding organs is also often carried out (Table VI). Death directly due to curative operation was 2.6%; 2.2% for distal gastrectomy and 3.7% for total gastrectomy (Table IV). Table V shows the long-term results of curative operation

TABLE III. Periodic Variation in 5-Year Survival Rate after Radical Operation
(Solitary Cancer; Curative Cases)

| Period | 5-Year survival rate (%) | | |
	Early cancer	Advanced cancer	Total curative cases
1946–1950	100.0 (1/1)	39.0 (78/200)	39.3 (79/201)
1951–1955	87.5 (21/24)	38.0 (208/548)	40.0 (229/572)
1956–1960	88.1 (59/67)	38.5 (284/739)	42.5 (343/806)
1961–1965	89.9 (134/149)	46.2 (289/626)	54.6 (423/775)
1966–1970	91.7 (209/228)	45.8 (258/563)	59.0 (467/791)
Total	90.4 (424/469)	41.8 (1,117/2,676)	49.0 (1,541/3,145)

TABLE IV. Curative Operation Technique and Operative Death Rate
(1946–1970; Solitary Cancer, Curative Cases)

| Operative technique | No. given radical operation | Operative death | |
		No. of cases	%
Distal gastrectomy	2,212	49	2.2
Total gastrectomy	827	31	3.7
Proximal gastrectomy	106	2	1.9
Total	3,145	82	2.6

TABLE V. Changes in Surgical Technique and 5-Year Survival
(Solitary Cancer ; Curative Casese)

Period	Distal gastrectomy			Total gastrectomy			Proximal gastrectomy		
	Actual		Relative	Actual		Relative	Actual		Relative
1946–1950	42	(70/168)	45	30	(9/30)	32	0	(0/3)	
1951–1955	48	(185/385)	53	23	(43/185)	25	50	(1/2)	64
1956–1960	49	(272/553)	55	27	(65/240)	30	46	(6/13)	53
1961–1965	63	(339/539)	79	36	(75/207)	40	31	(9/29)	37
1966–1970	70	(395/567)	79	30	(49/165)	33	40	(23/59)	47
Total	57	(1,261/2,212)	64	29	(241/827)	32	38	(39/106)	43

Actual, actual 5-year survival rate (%) ; relative, relative survival rate (%).

TABLE VI. Surgical Technique for Combined Resection of Adjacent Organs, Operative
Death, and 5-Year Survival Rate (1946–1970 ; Solitary Cancer, Curative Cases)

Technique	Operative death (%)	5-Year survival rate (%)
Thoracotomy-esophagectomy	5.9 (10/170)	17.6 (30/170)
Hepatectomy	6.7 (4/60)	33.3 (20/60)
Pancreatosplenectomy	3.4 (21/609)	24.6 (150/609)
Transverse resection of pancreas	3.0 (1/33)	33.3 (11/33)
Pancreatoduodenectomy	5.9 (7/119)	5.0 (6/119)
Colon resection	5.3 (17/318)	23.9 (76/318)
Total	4.4 (45/1,026)	24.9 (255/1,026)

according to surgical technique. The relative 5-year survival rate was 64% for distal gastrectomy and 32% for total gastrectomy. The 10-year survival rates were 44% (718/1,645) for distal gastrectomy, 20% (132/662) for total gastrectomy, and 30% (14/47) for proximal gastrectomy. The 5-year survival rate for distal gastrectomy was over 70% after 1961 but there was no improvement in the rate for total gastrectomy. The number of proximal gastrectomies is small, being 3.4% of all curative operations and its relative 5-year survival rate is 43%. Diagnosis of cancer in the upper part of the stomach has been difficult and many of the cases were in an advanced stage. With the progress in diagnostic technique, cases in an early stage should be operated upon so as to improve the 5-year survival rate for proximal gastrectomy to the level of that for distal gastrectomy.

For the infiltration of gastric cancer into surrounding organs and metastases to lymph nodes, combined resection of adjacent organs is being carried out (4). In spite of the complicated surgical technique required for combined resection with resection of the gastric lesion, direct death from the operation has been 4.4%, as shown in Table VI. The direct death rate was 5.9% when thoracotomy was combined to resect the esophagus, while it was 5.9% in the cases given combined pancreatoduodenectomy and 3.4% in combined pancreatosplenectomy. The 5-year survival rate in cases given combined resection is 25%, and it was 33% in cases given liver resection and transverse resection of the pancreas. There have been a large number of cases of pancreatosplenectomy and colectomy among combined resections, their relative 5-year survival rates being 25% and 24%. The majority of pancreatosplenectomies are combined with total gastrectomy, and the technique of combining pancreatosplenectomy with total gastrectomy is considered to be the typical technique for radical operation in advanced cancer present in the upper and middle portion of the stomach. The 5-year survival rate is 5% in cases given the combined pancreatoduodenectomy.

Factors Affecting Long-term Results

1. Sex and age

Relative 5-year survival rates according to sex are shown in Table VII. There is no difference between males and females, and there has been an improvement in the rate since 1961. Table VIII shows the 5-year survival rates according to age. In cases over 60 years of age, the actual 5-year survival rate is lower than that in other age groups but there is no difference in the relative survival rate. In young persons in their 20's and 30's, the relative 5-year survival rate is over 50%. It has been said that prognosis of gastric cancer in the younger age groups is poor but, according to our results limited to curative surgery, the relative 5-year survival rate is not different from that in other age groups.

TABLE VII. Five-year Survival Rate by Sex (Solitary Cancer ; Curative Cases)

Period	Males		Females	
	Actual	Relative	Actual	Relative
1946–1950	39 (50/127)	43	39 (29/74)	42
1951–1955	37 (134/364)	46	46 (95/208)	50
1956–1960	42 (210/502)	47	44 (133/304)	48
1961–1965	50 (232/466)	57	62 (191/309)	66
1966–1970	61 (297/484)	71	55 (169/307)	59
Total	48 (923/1,943)	54	51 (617/1,202)	56

Actual, actual 5-year survival rate (%) ; relative, relative 5-year survival rate (%).

2. Site of cancer

For the determination of the site of the central part of cancer, the stomach was divided into three parts, the upper (C), middle (M), and lower (A) portions according to the rules of the Japanese Research Society for Gastric Cancer (*1*). Table IX shows the 5-year survival rates according to the site of cancer; relative 5-year survival rates for cases with cancer in the middle and lower portions are 61% and 54%, respectively, which are better than that for cancer in the upper stomach. This survival rate has improved to over 60% for cases with cancer in the middle and lower part of the stomach since 1961 but, for cancer in the upper part of the stomach, improvement in prognosis has been small, the relative 5-year survival rate being 50% since 1965.

3. Macroscopic classification

When gastric cancer is limited to the mucosa and submucosa, they are classified as superficial cancer (the so-called early cancer). Advanced cancer is classified into 3 types macroscopically; the localized type, intermediate type, and infiltrative type (*2*). The localized type of cancer proliferates chiefly by expansion and the border with

TABLE VIII. Changes in 5-Year Survival Rate

| Period | Age | | | | | |
| | -29 | | 30-39 | | 40-49 | |
	Actual	Relative	Actual	Relative	Actual	Relative
1946–1950	33 (1/3)	34	48 (10/21)	49	40 (29/72)	42
1951–1955	75 (3/4)	76	61 (30/49)	62	47 (56/119)	49
1956–1960	43 (6/14)	43	51 (28/55)	52	50 (88/176)	51
1961–1965	69 (9/13)	70	67 (45/67)	68	66 (91/138)	68
1966–1970	46 (5/11)	46	59 (44/75)	59	74 (108/146)	77
Total	53 (24/45)	54	59 (157/267)	60	57 (372/651)	60

Actual, actual 5-year survival rate (%); relative 5-year survival rate (%).

TABLE IX. Five-year Survival Rate and Site of Cancer
(Solitary Cancer; Curative Cases)

| Period | Site | | | | | |
| | A | | M | | C | |
	Actual	Relative	Actual	Relative	Actual	Relative
1946–1950	38 (56/148)	42	46 (20/44)	49	33 (3/9)	35
1951–1955	42 (168/402)	46	43 (50/117)	47	21 (11/53)	22
1956–1960	43 (202/470)	48	45 (114/251)	51	32 (27/85)	35
1961–1965	56 (210/373)	63	60 (177/294)	67	37 (36/98)	38
1966–1970	61 (224/369)	68	64 (186/291)	72	43 (56/131)	50
Total	49 (865/1,762)	54	55 (547/997)	61	35 (134/376)	39

Actual, actual 5-year survival rate (%); relative, relative 5-year survival rate (%).

the surrounding tissue is distinct. This corresponds approximately with the Borrmann types I and II. The infiltrative type proliferates into the surrounding tissue by infiltration or diffusion and the border with surrounding tissue is indistinct. An intermediate between these 2 types, which cannot be classified as either, is the intermediate type. These types are finally determined on the cut surface after Formalin fixation. We have already reported (5) the great significance of this macroscopic classification, especially that of the localized type, on clinical and prognostic results.

The localized type of cancer occupies 36% (953/2,676) of all curative advanced cancer and its prognosis is good, the relative 5-year survival rate being 62%. Infiltrative cancer accounts for 49% (1,320/2,676) of curative advanced cancers but prognosis is poor, the relative survival rate being 37% (Table X). The good prognosis of the localized type of cancer is due not only to the absence of infiltrative growth into the surrounding tissue but also to little metastasis, especially to less peritoneal dissemination, and the indications for surgery on the localized type of cancer should be widened aggressively.

Cases with superficial cancer (the so-called early cancer) have a good prognosis and their relative 5-year survival rate is 99%, but 25 cases of superficial cancer that died within 5 years after operation comprise 10% of all superficial cancers. We have examined the cause of death in the cases that died within 5 years (15) and found 1.3%

with Age (Solitary Cancer, Curative Cases)

(years)					
50–59		60–69		70–	
Actual	Relative	Actual	Relative	Actual	Relative
39 (27/70)	42	35 (12/34)	43	0 (0/1)	
40 (99/250)	43	28 (38/136)	33	23 (3/13)	33
45 (119/263)	50	35 (86/249)	42	33 (16/49)	49
53 (130/246)	56	47 (124/263)	56	50 (24/48)	77
63 (149/236)	67	55 (126/230)	64	38 (35/93)	59
49 (524/1,065)	53	42 (386/912)	51	38 (78/204)	59

TABLE X. Macroscopic Classification of Gastric Cancer and Changes in 5-Year Survival Rate (Solitary Cancer; Curative Cases)

Period	Superficial cancer		Localized type		Intermediate type		Infiltrative type	
	Actual	Relative	Actual	Relative	Actual	Relative	Actual	Relative
1946–1950	100 (1/1)	100	57 (41/72)	63	21 (6/28)	23	31 (31/100)	34
1951–1955	88 (21/24)	94	57 (115/203)	63	37 (27/73)	41	24 (66/272)	26
1956–1960	88 (59/67)	97	49 (142/287)	56	28 (26/93)	32	32 (116/359)	35
1961–1965	90 (134/149)	99	58 (127/218)	66	44 (48/108)	49	38 (114/300)	42
1966–1970	92 (209/228)	100	56 (97/173)	66	43 (43/101)	48	41 (118/289)	45
Total	90 (424/469)	99	55 (522/953)	62	37 (150/403)	42	34 (445/1,320)	37

Actual, actual 5-year survival rate (%); relative, relative 5-year survival rate (%).

due to direct death, 4.4% due to recurrence, 5.0% from other diseases, and 0.3% from unknown causes. Examination of the relationship between the presence or absence of lymph node metastasis in superficial cancer and recurrence showed that recurrence was greater in the metastasis-positive cases which comprised 18% of superficial cancers. Therefore, radical dissection of secondary lymph nodes is necessary even in superficial cancer.

4. Depth of invasion to gastric wall

The depth of invasion of cancer into the gastric wall has a great effect on the prognosis of gastric cancer. This depth of invasion is classified by histological examination into m, sm, pm, ss, and s, indicating that cancer has invaded the mucosa, submucosa, proper muscle, subserosa, and serosa, respectively. Serosal invasion is divided into s_0 (nonserosal invasion), s_1 (minimal invasion), s_2 (definite invasion), and s_3 (invasion into adjacent organs). In the cases with cancer confined to m and sm, the relative 5-year survival rates are 103% and 96%, respectively, while that in pm is 79% and that in ss is 57%, the prognosis being poor for cancer with serosal invasion (Table XI).

5. Lymph node metastasis

Regional lymph nodes of the stomach are classified into 16 by the rules of the Japanese Research Society for Gastric Cancer, and are divided into the four groups

TABLE XI. Depth of Invasion of Gastric Cancer and Changes

Period	m		sm		pm	
	Actual	Relative	Actual	Relative	Actual	Relative
1946–1950			100 (1/1)	103	82 (23/28)	90
1951–1955	100 (5/5)	108	84 (16/19)	91	62 (61/99)	68
1956–1960	95 (19/20)	102	85 (40/47)	92	70 (63/90)	77
1961–1965	96 (66/69)	103	86 (69/80)	96	75 (46/61)	86
1966–1970	92 (110/119)	103	90 (97/108)	99	81 (63/78)	87
Total	94 (200/213)	103	87 (223/255)	96	72 (256/356)	79

Actual, actual 5-year survival rate (%); relative, relative 5-year survival rate (%).

TABLE XII. Lymph Node Metastasis and Changes in

Period	n_0		n_1	
	Actual	Relative	Actual	Relative
1946–1950	68 (34/50)	76	44 (27/62)	47
1951–1955	69 (93/134)	76	48 (89/187)	53
1956–1960	77 (153/199)	86	47 (111/238)	53
1961–1965	83 (232/280)	91	62 (111/180)	69
1966–1970	85 (301/353)	95	60 (117/196)	69
Total	80 (813/1,016)	89	53 (455/863)	59

Actual, actual 5-year survival rate (%); relative, relative 5-year survival rate (%).

of n_1, n_2, n_3, and n_4 according to the sites (A, M, and C) occupied by cancer (*1*). The relationship between lymph node metastasis and 5-year survival is summarized in Table XII. The prognosis is good for the group without lymph node metastasis (n_0), its 5-year survival rate being 89%. The prognosis becomes progressively poorer as the cancer in the lymph node metastases advances from n_1 to n_2, n_3, and n_4. The degree of lymph node metastases has shown a change with time, cases with n_0 and n_1 increasing since 1961.

6. Classification by stages

Table XIII shows the prognosis of cancer according to clinical stages as classified by the Japanese Research Society for Gastric Cancer (*1*). This staging is based chiefly on the serosal invasion of cancer and progress of lymph node metastasis. The prognosis of gastric cancer corresponds well with the progress in stages.

In cases of gastric cancer with liver metastasis, peritoneal dissemination and remote lymph node metastasis (especially to the para-aortic lymph node), for which radical operation is not indicated, we have carried out the dissection of remote metastasis; there were 10 cases that lived for 5 years or more. Details of these cases are shown in Table XIV, and included 6 of 83 cases with dissection of positive para-aortic lymph node metastasis (*10*), 2 cases with wedge-type resection of a solitary small metastatic focus limited to the left hepatic lobe, and 2 cases with dissection of the metastatic focus in the Douglas pouch. This fact indicates that, in metastasis of a localized type of gastric cancer to the para-aortic lymph node, aggressive dissection would allow in 5-Year Survival Rate (Solitary Cancer ; Curative Cases)

ss		s_1		s_2		s_3	
Actual	Relative	Actual	Relative	Actual	Relative	Actual	Relative
41 (27/66)	45	47 (15/32)	51	20 (12/61)	21	8 (1/13)	8
44 (97/221)	50	37 (27/73)	42	19 (20/104)	21	6 (3/51)	6
47 (173/367)	53	37 (27/74)	42	17 (17/103)	18	4 (4/105)	4
57 (132/233)	63	48 (67/140)	54	30 (42/141)	33	4 (2/51)	4
66 (91/137)	77	45 (64/141)	52	25 (35/138)	29	6 (4/68)	10
51 (520/1,024)	57	43 (200/460)	49	23 (127/547)	25	5 (14/288)	5

5-Year Survival Rate (Solitary Cancer ; Curative Cases)

n_2		n_3		n_4	
Actual	Relative	Actual	Relative	Actual	Relative
22 (17/78)	23	10 (1/10)	11	0 (0/1)	
21 (40/193)	23	9 (4/47)	10	0 (0/11)	
27 (78/290)	30	5 (3/66)	5	8 (1/13)	9
30 (69/233)	33	16 (10/64)	17	6 (1/18)	6
25 (43/173)	28	11 (6/53)	13	0 (0/16)	
26 (247/967)	28	10 (24/240)	12	3 (2/59)	4

TABLE XIII. Five-year Survival Rate According to Stages
(Solitary Cancer ; Curative Cases)

Period	Stage							
	I		II		III		IV	
	Actual	Relative	Actual	Relative	Actual	Relative	Actual	Relative
1946–1950	74 (20/27)	81	46 (34/74)	50	27 (24/90)	29	10 (1/10)	11
1951–1955	90 (60/67)	98	54 (123/226)	60	19 (43/221)	21	5 (3/59)	5
1956–1960	88 (119/136)	98	48 (192/399)	54	14 (29/202)	16	4 (3/71)	5
1961–1965	89 (185/208)	100	59 (158/268)	66	33 (74/223)	37	8 (6/74)	9
1966–1970	91 (262/287)	102	62 (152/245)	71	27 (45/168)	31	9 (8/90)	10
Total	89 (646/725)	99	54 (659/1,212)	61	24 (215/904)	26	7 (21/304)	8

Actual, actual 5-year survival rate (%) ; relative, relative 5-year survival rate (%).

some cases to survive for 5 years or more, as long as there was no factor(s) that might contraindicate radical surgery.

CONCLUSIONS

Examination of the therapeutic results for gastric cancer in the Department of Surgery, Cancer Institute Hospital, Tokyo, has revealed that the marked improvement in therapeutic results in the 1960's is primarily due to the increased number of cases

T. KAJITANI AND K. TAKAGI

TABLE XIV. Five-year Survival Cases of Gastric Cancer

Patient No.	Record No.	Age and Sex (years)	Cancer[a] site	Macroscopic type	S	P	H	n
1	290–60	58 ♂	CME	Localized	S_1	P_0	H_0	n_4
2	178–60	46 ♀	A	Localized	S_1	P_0	H_0	n_4
3	347–62	70 ♂	MA	Localized	S_1	P_0	H_0	n_4
4	465–64	57 ♂	M	Intermediate	S_0	P_0	H_0	n_4
5	497–64	50 ♂	MA	Localized	S_0	P_0	H_0	n_4
6	325–66	58 ♀	Mc	Localized	S_1	P_1	H_0	n_4
7	94–62	59 ♀	Mc	Intermediate	S_1	P_2	H_0	n_2
8	270–63	49 ♂	AM	Intermediate	S_1	P_2	H_0	n_1
9	626–58	66 ♂	A	Intermediate	S_2	P_0	H_1	n_2
10	769–70	73 ♀	Cm	Intermediate	S_2	P_0	H_1	n_2

[a] A, lower part of stomach ; M, middle part of stomach ; C, upper part of stomach.

[b] PS, pancreatosplenectomy ; TRP, transverse resection of pancreas.

with early cancer owing to the progress in stomach cancer diagnosis. This fact indicates the importance of early detection of gastric cancer for improving the therapeutic results of the disease. Even in advanced cases, in which cancer has infiltrated the proper muscle or deeper, it became possible to obtain a 42% 5-year survival rate by carrying out aggressive radical surgery with judgment of the macroscopic type of cancer, confirmation of the progress of cancer, selection of surgical technique, and especially with combined resection of adjacent organs with exhaustive dissection of lymph nodes.

It is not rare, nowadays, to find improvement in the long-term results by adjuvant chemotherapy but treatment of gastric cancer has been by radical gastrectomy. As has been iterated above, total gastrectomy cases have increased from the 1950's and dissection of regional lymph nodes has been extended to the limit, but death directly due to curative operation has lowered to 3.7%, indicating that there is no danger from the surgical treatment. Curability by surgical operation seems to have reached a limit with respect to gastric cancer.

We have described the therapeutic results of gastric cancer in the 1960's, and we await with interest what improvements will be brought about in the 1970's in diagnosis, surgical technique, and combined chemotherapy for the treatment of gastric cancer.

REFERENCES

1. Japanese Research Society for Gastric Cancer. *In* "General Rules for Castric Cancer Study in Surgery and Pathology," 9th Ed., Kanehara Shuppan, Tokyo (1974) (in Japanese).
2. Kajitani, T. Clinical classification of gastric cancer and its significance. *Gann*, **41**, 76–77 (1950).
3. Kajitani, T. Results of surgical treatment of gastric cancer. *GANN Monogr.*, **3**, 245–251 (1968).

Patients without Indication for Curative Surgical Operation

Surgical technique[b]	Chemotherapy[c]		Remarks
Total gastrectomy+PS	None		Out of n_4, one para-aortic lymph node removed
Gastrectomy+TRP	None		Out of n_4, two para-aortic lymph nodes removed
Gastretomy	MMC Ex	60 mg 129 g	Out of n_4, para-aortic lymph node and Virchow's lymph node removed
Gastretomy	MMC	40 mg	Out of n_4, two para-aortic lymph nodes removed
Gastretomy	MMC	40 mg	Out of n_4, two para-aortic lymph nodes removed
Total gastrectomy+PS +liver resection	MMC	28 mg	P_1 is a contact metastasis to left lobe of liver. Out of n_4, 5 para-aortic lymph node removed
Total gastrectomy+PS	MMC	34 mg	Out of P_2, one bean-sized metastasis in Douglas pouch removed
Gastretomy	MMC	40 mg	Two grain-sized metastases (P_2) in Douglas pouch removed
Gastrectomy+liver resection	None		Wedge resection of one fingertip-sized H_1 in left lobe of liver
Total gastrectomy+PS +liver resection	None		One bean-sized H_1 in left lobe of liver resected

[c] MMC, Mitomycin-C ; Ex, Endoxan.

S, serosal invasion ; P, peritoneal dissemination ; H, liver metastasis ; n, lymph node metastasis.

4. Kajitani, T. and Nishi, M. Combined operation of gastric cancer and its selection. *Geka (Surgery)*, **29**, 1369–1381 (1967) (in Japanese).

5. Kajitani, T. Gastric cancer. *In* "Modern Surgery," Nakayama Shoten, Tokyo, Vol. 35B, pp. 20–26 (1971) (in Japanese).

6. Kurokawa, T., Kajitani, T., and Oota, K. "Carcinoma of the Stomach in Early Phase," Nakayama Shoten, Tokyo (1966).

7. Kuru, M. "Atlas of Early Gastric Cancer," Nakayama Shoten, Tokyo (1966).

8. Muto, M. "Gastric Cancer Observed from Surgical Side," Kanehara Shuppan, Tokyo (1963) (in Japanese).

9. Nakayama, K., Yanagisawa, H., Honma, Y., and Matsuno, N. Prognosis of gastric cancer operation. *Sogo Rinsho (Clinic All-Round)*, **9**, 1061–1070 (1960) (in Japanese).

10. Ohashi, I., Takagi, K., Konishi, T., Izumoi, S., Fukami, A., and Kajitani, T. Five-year survival cases with dissection of para-aortic lymph-node metastases from gastric cancer. *Nippon Shokaki Geka Gakkaishi (Japan. J. Gastroenterol. Surg.)*, **9**, 112–116 (1976) (in Japanese).

11. Sakita, T. and Oguro, Y. Routine gastrocamera examination. *GANN Monogr. Cancer Res.*, **11**, 145–157 (1971).

12. Segi, M. and Kurihara, N. "Cancer Mortality for Selected Sites in 24 Countries, No. 5, 1964–65," Tohoku University School of Medicine, Sendai (1969).

13. Shirakabe, H., Ichikawa, H., Kumakura, K., Nishizawa, M., Higurashi, K., Hayakawa, H., and Murakami, T. "Atlas of X-ray Diagnosis of Early Gastric Cancer," Igaku Shoin, Tokyo (1966).

14. Takagi, K. Diagnosis of early gastric cancer by fibergastroscopic biopsy. *In* "Endoscopy of the Digestive System," Proc. 1st European Congr. of Digestive Endoscopy, Prague, Karger, Basel/New York, pp. 67–69 (1969).

15. Takagi, K. and Nakada, K. Lymph-node metastases and surgical results on early gastric cancer. *Rinsho Geka (Clinical Surgery)*, **31**, 19–27 (1976) (in Japanese).

CANCER OF THE COLON AND RECTUM

Dennosuke Jinnai and Masayuki Yasutomi

*Department of Surgery, Kinki University School of Medicine**

Out of a total of 485 cases of cancer of the large intestine, 143 had cancer of the colon and 342 cancer of the rectum. Curative resection was performed on 376 (or 77.5%) of the patients, and the operative death rate was 2.4% (9 cases). The 5-year survival rates were 73.3% for cancer of the colon and 55.9% for cancer of the rectum, giving an overall rate of 60.7%. The relative survival rates obtained from the Japanese Life Table were 82.5%, 60.1%, and 66.1%, respectively. There have been major changes in the operative methods for rectal cancer since 1962. The trend has been to perform sphincter preserving operations whenever possible in place of Miles operations which were most common before 1961. Additionally the regional lymph nodes have been thoroughly dissected since 1962. As a result, sphincter preserving operations, which accounted for only 14.4% of the operations prior to 1961, have increased to 41.7% since 1962, and the absolute 5-year survival rates have also increased from 52.9 to 59.1%. Comparison of sphincter preserving and Miles operations for cancer at the same site and stage, showed that survival rates did not decrease with the sphincter preserving operations.

The results of the treatment of 208 cases of early rectal cancer collected from 10 institutions showed a 96.9% absolute 5-year survival rate.

It has been reported that the incidence of cancer of the large intestine in Japan has been increasing year by year during the last two decades, while it is still low compared to other countries (*10*). Special attention has been turned toward cancer of the large intestine from gastric cancer which has the highest incidence of any cancer in Japan. In 1973, the Japanese Research Society for Colon and Rectal Cancer (*4*) was established with a membership of more than 100 surgeons, physicians, radiologists, and pathologists in the medical schools and leading hospitals in Japan. This society, having detailed descriptive data for cancers of the colon and rectum, has set up a prescription and a terminology for use in the diagnosis, treatment, and recording of end results.

The progress in the field of X-ray examination and colonofiberscopy has focussed attention on the diagnosis and treatment of early cancer of the large intestine. Described in this paper is a statistical study of the cases of cancer of the large intestine treated by the authors at the Surgical Department of Osaka University Hospital during 1954–1975, as well as early cancers of the large intestine treated at 10 representative surgical clinics in Japan.

---

* Nishiyama 380, Sayama-cho, Minami Kawachi-gun, Osaka 589, Japan (陣内伝之助, 安富正幸).

Cancer of the Large Intestine as a Whole

From 1954 to 1975, 485 cases of primary cancer of the large intestine were admitted to the Surgical Department of Osaka University Hospital. Of these patients, 143 (34.8%) had cancer of the colon and 342 (65.2%) cancer of the rectum. Curative resection was performed on 376 (77.5%) out of the 485 cases. Among the 143 cases of cancer of the colon, 111 (77.6%) underwent the curative resection; there were 3 operative deaths (2.7%). Among the 342 cases of cancer of the rectum, 265 (77.5%) underwent curative resection and 6 died in the 30 postoperative days (operative death rate: 2.3%). The absolute 5-year survival rates following curative resection were 60.7% for cancer of the large intestine, 73.7% for cancer of the colon, and 55.9% for cancer of the rectum. The relative 5-year survival rates corrected for sex, age, and year were 66.1% for all curative cases, 82.5% for cancer of the colon, and 60.1% for cancer of the rectum (Table I). The age and sex distribution at the time of the operation is shown in Table II. The age of the patients varied from 21 to 84 years, with a mean of 57.9 years. Among the 485 cases of cancer of the large intestine, 306 (63.1%) were males and 179 (36.9%) were females. The male to female ratio was 1.7: 1.

Curative resection was performed on 78.1% of the males and 76.0% of the females. According to the macroscopic classification of the primary tumor by the Japanese Research Society for Colon and Rectal Cancer, 16.5% of the cases were circumscribed tumorous cancer, 61.9% were circumscribed ulcerous cancer, 20.4% were infiltrating

TABLE I. Results of Treatment of Cancer of the Colon and Rectum (1954–1975)

Site of lesion	Number of primary cases admitted	Number of curative resections (%)	Number of operative deaths (%)	Lived 5 or more years	5-Year survival rates	
					Absolute (%)	Relative (%)
Rectum	143	111 (77.6)	3 (2.7)	56/76	73.7	82.5
Colon	342	265 (77.5)	6 (2.3)	114/204	55.9	60.1
Total	485	376 (77.5)	9 (2.4)	170/280	60.7	66.1

TABLE II. Age and Sex Distribution of Patients with Cancer of the Large Intestine

Age (years)	Cancer of the rectum		Cancer of the colon		Cancer of the large intestine		Total number
	Male	Female	Male	Female	Male	Female	
20–	13 (7)	6 (2)	2 (1)	2 (1)	15 (8)	8 (3)	23 (11)
30–	30 (25)	22 (17)	5 (5)	1 (0)	35 (30)	23 (17)	58 (47)
40–	15 (11)	28 (20)	17 (13)	9 (7)	32 (24)	37 (27)	69 (51)
50–	59 (49)	31 (25)	22 (17)	16 (12)	81 (66)	47 (37)	128 (103)
60–	60 (49)	31 (26)	30 (25)	11 (8)	90 (74)	42 (34)	132 (108)
70–	34 (24)	11 (8)	17 (11)	11 (10)	51 (35)	22 (18)	73 (53)
80–	2 (2)	0 (0)	0 (0)	0 (0)	2 (2)	0 (0)	2 (2)
Total number	213 (167)	129 (98)	93 (72)	50 (38)	306 (239)	179 (136)	485 (375)
	342 (265)		143 (110)				

( ) Number of curative resections.

ulcerous cancer, and 1.1% were diffuse infiltrating cancer. Histologically, 86% of the cases were well or moderately differentiated adenocarcinoma. Usually, cancers of the large intestine were separated into those originating in the colon and those originating in the rectum, because there are definite differences between these cancers in terms of the surgical procedures involved, prognosis, and postoperative functions.

1. Cancer of the rectum

Among 342 cases of cancer of the rectum, there were 135 cases (39.5%) of cancers of the rectosigmoid and the upper rectum, which were collected above the peritoneal reflection, 181 cases (52.9%) of cancer of the lower rectum, and 26 cases (7.6%) of cancer of the anal canal, from the upper margin of the puborectal muscle to the anal verge. Of all of these patients, 265 underwent curative resection (77.5% curative resection rate): 110 cases (or 81.5%) with cancer above the peritoneal reflection; 135 cases (or 74.6%) of the lower rectum, and 20 cases (or 76.9%) of the anal canal underwent curative resection (Table III). Radical procedures employed in treating cancer of the rectum are shown in Table IV, which include Miles abdominoperineal resection in 181 cases, anterior resection in 38, pull-through operation (2, 5) in 29, the invagination procedure (11) in 6, and local excision in 11. From 1954 to 1961 Miles operations were performed in almost all cases of cancer of the rectum. After 1962, however, sphincter preserving operations such as anterior resections, invagination procedures, and pull-through operations were performed readily. Among curative resections prior to 1961, 83 (85.6%) were by Miles operation and only 14 (14.7%) were by sphincter preserving operations, and among the latter 14 cases, 10 were anterior resections for cancer in the rectosigmoid. Since 1962, however, Miles operation has accounted for 98 (58.3%) of

TABLE III. Results of Treatment of Cancer of the Rectum According to Site (1954–1975)

Site of primary tumor	Admitted cases	Number of curative resections (%)	5-Year absolute survivals (%)
Upper rectum (including rectosigmoid)	135	110 (81.5)	53/85 (62.3)
Lower rectum	181	135 (74.6)	53/104 (51.0)
Anal canal	26	20 (76.9)	8/15 (53.5)
Total	342	265 (77.5)	114/204 (55.9)

TABLE IV. Radical Procedures Employed in Treating Cancer of the Rectum

Procedures	Number of cases		Total number of cases (%)
	1954–1961 (%)	1962–1975 (%)	
Miles operation	83[a]* (85.6)	98[b]* (58.3)	181 (68.2)
Pull-through operation	1 (1.0)	28 (16.7)	29 (11.0)
Invagination procedure	0	6 (3.6)	6 (2.3)
Anterior resection	10 (10.5)	28 (16.7)	38 (14.3)
Local excision	3 (3.1)	8 (4.8)	11 (4.2)
Total	97 (100)	168 (100)	265 (100)

[a] Including 2 cases of Hartmann's operation.   * p<0.01
[b] Including 3 cases of pelvic exenteration.

TABLE V. Radical Procedures Employed for Cancer of the Rectosigmoid
and the Upper Rectum (1954–1975)

Procedures	Number of cases		Total (%)
	1954–1961 (%)	1962–1970 (%)	
Miles operation	20 (64.5)*	23 (29.1)*	43 (39.0)
Pull-through operation	0 (0)	17 (21.5)	17 (15.5)
Invagination procedure	0 (0)	5 (6.3)	5 (4.5)
Anterior resection	10 (32.3)	28 (35.4)	38 (34.5)
Local excision	1 (3.2)	6 (7.6)	7 (6.4)
Total	31 (100)	79 (100)	110 (100)

* $p < 0.01$

the 168 curative resections. The remaining 60 (41.7%) underwent sphincter preserving operations (Table IV).

As shown in Table V, among the curative resections of cancer of the rectosigmoid and the upper rectum, only 29.1% were treated with Miles operations while 70.9% were with sphincter preserving operations. Prior to 1961, however, Miles operations accounted for 64.5% and sphincter preserving operations for 35.5%. Almost all of the cancers of the lower rectum and anal canal were given Miles operations through the entire term from 1954 to 1975. Prior to 1961, Miles operation was considered obligatory as the radical procedure for rectal cancer. From 1962 to 1975, however, sphincter preserving operations were almost universally administered for cancer of the rectosigmoid and the upper rectum, and Miles operations were performed for cancer of the lower rectum and anal canal.

The survival rates have proved to be dependent upon many factors such as the size and type of tumor, its location, the grade of mural depth invasion, particularly, whether it has infiltrated or adhered to adjacent tissue or not, the age and sex of the patient, and the type and extent of operative procedures performed. Of the 204 patients who underwent curative resections for cancer of the rectum during 1954–1970, 114 cases (or 55.9%) survived at least 5 years, but the rate in the group during 1962–1970 was considerably better, this being 59.1% as compared to 52.1% for the former group from 1954 to 1961 (Table VI). Of 85 cases of cancer of the rectosigmoid and the upper rectum during 1954–1970, 53 cases (or 62.3%) survived 5 years or more, and their survival rates were composed of 51.5% prior to 1961 and 68.5% after 1962. It is interesting to note that the statistically significant improvement in the 5-year survival rate was

TABLE VI. Five-year Survivals after Curative Resection for Cancer of Rectum (1954–1970)

Procedures	Number of cases		Total (%)
	1954–1961 (%)	1962–1975 (%)	
Miles operation	41/81 (50.6)	32/65 (49.2)	73/146 (50.0)
Pull-through operation	1/1	11/20 (55.0)	12/21 (57.1)
Invagination procedure	0	3/3	3/3
Anterior resection	5/10 (50.0)	15/18 (83.3)	20/28 (71.4)
Local excision	2/2	4/4	6/6
Total	49/94 (52.1)	65/110 (59.1)	114/204 (55.9)

TABLE VII. Five-year Survivals after Curative Resection for Cancer
of the Rectosigmoid and the Upper Rectum (1954–1970)

Procedures	Number of cases		Total (%)
	1954–1961 (%)	1962–1970 (%)	
Miles operation	10/20 (50.0)	8/18 (44.4)	18/38 (47.4)
Pull-through operation	0	8/12 (66.7)	8/12 (66.7)
Invagination procedure	0	3/3 (100)	3/3 (100)
Anterior resection	5/10 (50.0)	15/18 (83.3)	20/28 (71.4)
Local excision	1/1 (100)	3/3 (100)	4/4 (100)
Total	16/31 (51.5)*	37/54 (68.5)*	53/85 (62.3)

* $p < 0.01$

observed after 1962 when the sphincter preserving operations were performed on the basis of a strict indication (Table VII). Fifty-three (51.0%) of lower rectum cases and 8 (53.0%) of 15 anal cases lived 5 years or more. It is thought that these improvements in the treatment of cancer of the rectosigmoid and the upper rectum after 1962, that is, more than of 70% curative resections were sphincter preserving operations as shown in Table V and the 5-year survival rate attained 68.5% as shown in Table VII, depended mainly upon a properly selected sphincter preserving operation and adequate removal of the primary lesion as well as the associated tissues containing regional lymphatics. As concerns the dissection of the regional lymph nodes, inferior mesenteric and superior rectal nodes were removed completely for all rectal cancers, and besides, the middle rectal nodes, internal iliac nodes, obturator nodes, middle sacral nodes, and inferior rectal nodes were dissected for Dukes B and C cancer of the lower rectum and anal canal. There were no significant increases, however, through these two periods, in the 5-year survivals for cases of cancer of the lower rectum and anal canal. According to the Astler-Coller classification (1), the 5-year survival rates following curative resection for cancer of the rectum were 100% for Stage A, 75.0% for Stage B_1, 67.0% for Stage B_2, 52.1% for Stage C_1, and 45.0% for Stage C_2. In an analysis of comparable lesions under the Astler-Coller classification, the survival rates were almost equal in sphincter preserving operations and Miles operation for patients without lymph node involvement. That is, the 5-year survival rates were 100% for Astler-Coller's A of both groups, 75.0% for Stage B_1 of both groups, and 68.4% and 66.1%, respectively, for Stage B_2. In patients with lymph node involvement, however, survival rates from the Miles operation and sphincter preserving operation were 34.8% and 87.5%, respectively, for Stage C_1, and 28.8% and 54.5% for Stage C_2 (Table VIII). The overall 5-year survival rates after radical resection were 70.7% for sphincter preserving operations while being 50.0% for Miles operations. It would seem that sphincter preserving operations gave better results than the Miles operation, but these differences resulted from the fact that sphincter preserving operations were administered for cancers with less involvement of the lymph nodes and associated tissues. According to the macroscopic classification of tumors, proposed by the Japanese Research Society of Colon and Rectal Cancer (4), cancers of the colon and rectum are divided into the noninvasive type, circumscribed tumorous type, circumscribed ulcerous type, infiltrating ulcerous type, diffuse infiltrating type and unclassified type. The 5-year survival rates for cancer

TABLE VIII.   Five-year Survival Rates following Curative Resection for Cancer
of the Rectum: According to the Astler-Coller Classification

Astler-Coller classification	Miles operation (%)	Sphincter preserving operation (%)	Total (%)
A	100	100	100
B_1	75.0	75.0	75.0
B_2	66.1	68.4	67.0
C_1	34.8	87.5	52.1
C_2	28.8	54.5	45.0
Total	50.0	70.7	55.9

of the rectum from the macroscopic classification were as follows: 100% for non-invasive cancer, 72.2% for circumscribed tumorous cancer, 48.7% for circumscribed ulcerous cancer, 23.5% for infiltrating ulcerous cancer, and 0% for the 2 cases of diffuse infiltrating cancer. When cancer of the rectum was classified according to the size of tumor, the 5-year survival rates were 77.8% for those less than 2 cm in diameter, 63.6% for those less than 3 cm, 62.7% for those less than 5 cm, 47.8% for those less than 7 cm, and 33.3% for those 7 cm or more. The size of a tumor was partly significant in the prognosis of cancer of the rectum. The classification of the mural depths of the cancer invasion proposed by the Japanese Research Society was appraised as having prognostic value. There were mucosal cancer (m) in 4 cases, submucosal cancer (sm) in 7 cases, cancer which had infiltrated into the proper muscle layer (pm) in 69 cases, cancer which had penetrated slightly beyond the proper muscle layer (a_1) in 78 cases, cancer which had penetrated markedly beyond the proper muscle layer (a_2) in 66 cases, and cancer which had infiltrated into adjacent organs (a_i) in 36 cases. The 5-year survival rates from mural depth invasion were 100% for m and sm, 56.6% for pm, 47.5% for a_1, and 33.3% for a_2 and a_i.

Although the results of surgery were mainly discussed as afore-mentioned, there remains the important problem of fecal control after sphincter preserving operations in rectal surgery. The anal functions of patients who underwent anterior resection, invagination, and pull-through operations were examined. In anterior resection cases, excellent fecal control was kept intact even immediately after the operation, although all pull-through patients complained of a degree of fecal incontinence for up to about 3 months after operation. Fecal control of pull-through patients, however, showed gradual improvement and 2 years after surgery, only 32% of the patients complained of fecal control disturbances and about two-thirds had obtained fairly good control. Based upon the excellent results in fecal control of the invagination procedure, it is believed that normal anal functions will result from leaving the rectal stump extending 2–3 cm beyond the dentate line.

2.   Cancer of the colon

Cancer of the colon accounted for 143 (or 34.8%) of 485 cases for all cancers of the large intestine. There were 93 males and 50 females, yielding a male to female ratio of 1.9: 1. The youngest patient was 24 years old, the oldest 82. The mean age was 60.2 years, and the great majority of lesions occurred in those over 40 years of age. The highest incidence was in the sixties in males and in the fifties in females (Tables

I and II). Of the 143 afore-mentioned cancers, 20 were located in the cecum, 25 in the ascending colon, 27 in the transverse colon, 11 in the descending colon, and 60 in the sigmoid colon. Curative resections were performed in 111 of the 143 cases. The curative resection rates were 77.6% for all cancers of the colon: 76.2% for the right colon and 77.6% for the left colon, and 70.0% for the transverse colon. Three patients died within one month after curative resection (operative death rate: 2.7%). According to the standards adopted by the authors for radical colectomy of advanced cancer, removal of a tumor-bearing colon 10 cm or more from both sides of the tumor margins is recommended, including the epicolic, paracolic, intermediate, and main nodes. The most common procedures utilized for curative resections were right hemicolectomies for cancer in the right colon, and partial colectomies for cancer in the transverse and the left colon. Subtotal colectomies and left hemicolectomies were carried out only for about one-fourth of the patients in cancers of the left colon. The 5-year survival rates were 73.7% for all curative resections, 71.0% for cancer of the right colon, 78.5% for the transverse colon, and 75.8% for the left colon. Under the Astler-Coller classification, the absolute 5-year survival rates for curative resections during 1954–1970 were 73.7% for all cancers, 100% for A, 85.6% for B_1, 73.2% for B_2, 56.1% for C_1, and 46.1% for C_2. There was no significant correlation between the size of the primary tumor and 5-year survival rates, except that the survival rate was 100% for tumors less than 3 cm in diameter. There were no cases of survival over 5 years after non-curative operations.

Early Cancer of the Large Intestine

With the recent advances in the field of colonofiberscopic and radiographic examinations, it has become easy to detect early cancer of the large intestine in Japan. Early cancer of the large intestine has been defined as an intramucosal and submucosal cancer by the afore-mentioned Japanese Research Society of Colon and Rectal Cancer, this being the same definition as that for gastric cancer, and it was classified macroscopically into: I, protruded type; IIa, superficial elevated type; IIb, superficial flat type; IIc, superficial depressed type; and III, excavated type. The author found 21 cases of early cancer (or 4.3%) amongst the 485 cases of cancer of the large intestine. Local excision including polypectomy was performed in 7 of 21 cases and colectomy in 14 cases; all patients with early cancer remained alive 5 years or more. It is difficult, however, to evaluate the end results of early cancer treatment on the basis of only 21 early cancers. In order to obtain a large enough number of patients to understand the most proper surgical techniques to be used for early cancer of the large intestine, 208 cases of early cancer were collected from 10 representative surgical clinics in Japan. The 208 cases correspond to 6.1% of 3,424 cases with cancer of the large intestine in 10 clinics and were comprised of 102 cases of mucosal cancer (or 3.0%) and 106 cases of submucosal cancer (or 3.1%) (Table IX). The male to female ratio of the 208 patients was 1.6: 1. These early cancers were most often found in the rectum (71.7%) and in the sigmoid colon (24.3%) while only one case was in the right colon. The reason why early cancer in the right colon was scarcely detected might be the difficulty of diagnosing by radiographic and fiberscopic examinations. Macroscopically, the majority of early cancers were of the protruded type (type I: 77.9%), followed by the superficial

TABLE IX. Frequency of Early Cancer of the Large Intestine

Early cancer	m	sm	m+sm
	102 (3.0%)	106 (3.1%)	208 (6.1%)
Total cases of colon and rectal cancer		3,424	

m, mucosal cancer; sm, submucosal cancer.

TABLE X. Macroscopic Classification of Early Cancer in the Large Intestine

Classification				No. of cases	%	
I	protruded type	I_p	long pedunc.	66	33.2 } 57.8	77.9
			short pedunc.	49	24.6	
		I_s	sessile	40	20.1 } 20.1	
II_a	superficial elevated type			39	19.6	
II_c or III	superficial depressed and excavated type			5	2.5	

Excluding 9 cases of unclassified cancer.

elevated one (type IIa: 19.6%), and the excavated and superficial depressed type (types III and IIc: 2.5%) (Table X). Histologically, more than half of the lesions were papillary adenocarcinomas and the remaining ones were differentiated adenocarcinomas. There were no cases of hematogenous metastasis in the intramucosal cancers, three (2.9%) among the 101 cases of submucosal cancer, however, disclosed liver metastasis at the time of, or after operation. There were no cases of lymphatic metastasis among the intramucosal cancers, but it was found in 6 (5.7%) of 105 cases of submucosal cancer. The surgical procedures utilized for early cancers consist of 38 cases of polypectomy (18.3%), 20 cases of wedge resection (9.6%), and 150 cases of colectomy (72.1%) (Table XI). There were only a few cases of endoscopic polypectomy which

TABLE XI. Operative Procedures for Early Cancer of the Large Intestine

1.	Polypectomy	38 (18.3%)
2.	Wedge resection	20 (9.6%)
	Transanal	
	Trans-sphincteric (Mason)	
	Trans-sacral (Kraske)	
	Transabdominal	
3.	Colectomy	150 (72.1%)
	Total	208 (100%)

TABLE XII. Five-year Survival Rates of Early Cancer from Various Operative Procedures

Operative procedure	Number of cases	Number of survivals	5-Year survival rate (%)
Polypectomy	23	22	95.7
Wedge resection	7	7	100.0
Colectomy	97	94	96.9
Total	127	123	96.9

has become a common treatment for polypoid lesions in the colon and rectum in Japan since these 208 cases were collected from surgical clinics. In terms of long-term results concerning early cancers of the large intestine, it was found that patients lived 5 years or more in 94 (96.9%) of the 97 segmental resection cases and 22 (95.7%) of the 23 polypectomy cases. A total of 123 (96.9%) of 127 patients with early cancer remained alive 5 years or more without suffering a recurrence of the disease (Table XII).

DISCUSSION

According to information from the Japanese Ministry of Health and Welfare, there has been a definite increase in cancers of the colon and rectum during the last 25 years in Japan, and the age-adjusted mortality rate per 100,000 population has increased from 2.9 in 1947 to 6.9 in 1973, but the mortality rate is still one of the lowest in any country. During the 20 years following World War II, the dietary habits of the Japanese has changed strikingly. The consumption of eggs, milk, meat, fats, and fruits has increased 4 to 10 times according to the Japanese Ministry of Health and Welfare. It is suggested that there is an etiological relation between these dietary changes and the increment of cancer of the colon and rectum. The percentage distributions of colon and rectal cancer in Japan are different from those in Europe and the United States, that is, cancer of the rectum has a relatively higher distribution rate of 55–65% in Japan as against 50–60% in other countries. That more than 80% of colon and rectal cancers were of the circumscribed type in their gross appearance, well or moderately differentiated adenocarcinoma histologically, approximately 50% of which had no lymphatic involvement, was the reason why better results in the treatment of colon and rectal cancer were obtained compared to those of gastric cancer. The absolute 5-year survival rates in our series after curative resection were 73.7% for cancer of the colon and 55.9% for cancer of the rectum. Kajitani (1974) reported that a curative resection was performed for 79.0% of the 876 cases of colon and rectal cancer with absolute 5-year survival rates of 67.5% for cancer of the colon and 55.4% for cancer of the rectum. Although, in Japan, the frequency of colon and rectal cancer is low, there appears to have been an improvement in the survival rates in recent years. For cancer of the colon, a wider removal of the tumor-bearing colon through such procedures as hemicolectomies and subtotal colectomies with adequate dissection of the regional lymph nodes including the intermediate nodes and main nodes, has been performed. For cancer of the rectum, there have been some improvements and achievements during this 20-year period. The first is that there has been a distinct increase in the proportion of patients treated by means of sphincter preserving operations. From 1962 to 1975, more than 70% of the rectosigmoid and the upper rectum cancer cases were treated in this manner. In sphincter preserving operations, if a wider resection of the rectum were performed, the possibility of cancer recurrence might decrease, but more severe disturbances of fecal control would occur. On the contrary, if an insufficient resection of the rectum were performed, postoperative fecal control would be kept. Cancer, however, might recur at a high rate. An anterior resection consists of a transabdominal proctosigmoidectomy and re-established continuity by an end-to-end anastomosis. An invagination procedure consists of transabdominal proctosigmoidectomy leaving a rectal distal stump of 2 to 3 cm from the dentate line, and end-to-end anastomosis by which the oral colonic stump and the inverted rectal stump are joined outside the anus. In pull-through operation, the rectum is transected just above the dentate line, and after proctosigmoidectomy, the colonic stump is drawn through the anal canal, and anoplasty is performed 2 or 3 weeks later. The sphincter preserving operations are applicable for tumors the lower margin of which is 6 cm or more apart from the anal verge, and for tumors which are not intensely infiltrating to adjacent tissues or in a stage of advanced lymphatic involvement. Comparison of the Miles operation and sphincter preserving operation performed on the same sites and stages of cancer according to the Astler-Coller classification showed no decrease in the 5-year survival rates of the patients given the sphincter preserving operations. This indicates that there is sufficient curability when sphincter preserving operations are performed on the basis of appropriate selection and with adequate dissection of the regional lymph nodes. For Dukes C cancer situated in the lower rectum, Miles operation with complete abdominal and pelvic dissection including middle rectal, internal iliac, and obturator nodes in the lateral pedicle, middle and lateral sacral nodes in the posterior pedicle, and inferior mesenteric and superior rectal nodes in the superior pedicle with adequate removal of associated tissue should be applied. Early cancer of the large intestine, which was defined as mucosal and submucosal cancer by the Japanese Research Society of Colon and Rectal Cancer (4), accounted for 208 (or 6.1%) of 3,424 cases with cancer of the large intestine. Most of them (97.5%) were of the protruded or superficial elevated type in gross appearance and the majority (71.7%) were located in the rectum. These 208 cases were treated by colectomy (77.1%), polypectomy (18.3%), and wedge resection (9.6%), and their 5-year survival rate was 96.9%. It must be emphasized that polypectomy should not be applied except for pedunculated mucosal cancer (9), though wedge resection is used for carefully selected early cancer, because lymphatic metastases were formed in 5.7% of the submucosal cancers.

REFERENCES

1. Astler, V. B. and Coller, F. A. The prognostic significance of direct extension of carcinoma of the colon and rectum. *Ann. Surg.*, **139**, 846–851 (1954).
2. Bacon, H. E. "Cancer of the Colon, Rectum and Anal Canal," J. B. Lippincott, Co., Philadelphia (1964).
3. Enstrom, J. E. Colorectal cancer and consumption of beef and fat. *Br. J. Cancer*, **32**, 432–439 (1975).
4. Japanese Research Society for Colon and Rectal Cancer. "General Rules for Cancer of the Colon and Rectum" Kanehara Shuppan, Tokyo (1976) (in Japanese).
5. Jinnai, D. and Yasutomi, M. Sphincter preserving operation for the rectal cancer. *Nippon Gan Chiryo Gakkaishi* (*J. Japan. Soc. Cancer Ther.*), **7**, 191–203 (1972) (in Japanese).
6. Kajitani, T. and Takahashi, T. Problems in surgical treatments for cancer of the colon and rectum. *Igaku-no-Ayumi*, **94**, 600–605 (1976) (in Japanese).
7. Lockhart-Mummery, H. E., Ritchie, J. K., and Hawley, P. R. The results of surgical treatment for carcinoma of the rectum at St. Mark's Hospital from 1948 to 1972. *Br. J. Surg.*, **63**, 673–677 (1976).
8. Ministry of Health and Welfare of Japan. "The Present State of the Nutritional Intake of Japanese," Daiichi-shuppan, Tokyo, p. 39 (1976) (in Japanese).

9. Morson, B. C. Factors influencing the prognosis of early cancer of the rectum. *Proc. Roy. Soc. Med.*, **59**, 607–608 (1966).

10. Segi, M. and Kurihara, M. "Cancer Mortality for Selected Sites in 24 Countries. No. 6," Japan Cancer Society, Tokyo (1972).

11. Welch, C. S. and Rheinlander, H. F. Radical abdominal proctosigmoidectomy with preservation of the anal sphincter. *Surg. Gynecol. Obstet.*, **94**, 550–560 (1952).

GANN Monograph on Cancer Research 22, 1979

CANCER OF THE BLADDER

Hisao TAKAYASU and Kenkichi KOISO

Department of Urology, Faculty of Medicine, University of Tokyo*

A treatment and results in 123 patients with primary bladder cancer who visited the University of Tokyo Hospital between 1963 and 1969 are reviewed.

Many modes of surgical treatment of bladder cancer have been reported. However, in this hospital the treatment of bladder tumors is divided into four main categories: Transurethral resection (TUR); transurethral coagulation (TUC) of the bladder tumors; sectio alta with electroresection and coagulation, combined with or without radon-seed implantation; partial cystectomy, and cystectomy with urinary diversion. The decision about these therapeutic procedures depended mainly on extent of invasion of the tumors into the bladder wall (T classification), with reference to the surgical risks and the grades of the tumors (Broders), and other factors, such as the size, number and location.

The relative 5-year survival rates ($\pm 2\sigma r$) in each group were as follows: TUR, TUC: 0.887 ± 0.116, sectio alta+electroresection and coagulation: 0.747 ± 0.293, partial cystectomy: 0.571 ± 0.420, cystectomy (simple, radical): 0.450 ± 0.518.

Recurrences were higher in the partial cystectomy group than in other groups. The relative 5-year survival rates of the TUR, TUC, sectio alta, and partial cystectomy groups were almost the same as previously reported, while that of the cystectomy group was good.

Cancer of the bladder is the most important among the malignant tumors of the urinary tract. Many modes of treatment of bladder cancer have been reported; however, many problems remain unsolved.

This paper presents a review and results of treatment of bladder cancer by various surgical methods at the University of Tokyo Hospital between 1963 and 1969.

Patient Studies

1. Number of patients

From 1963 to 1969, 235 patients with primary bladder cancer visited our hospital. Of 235 patients 123 were followed-up until recently and subjected to this study. The remaining patients were sent to affiliated hospitals after the establishment of diagnosis.

2. Age and sex

The average age was 57.0 years; the range was 22 to 78 years. Sixty-three percent of the patients were between 50 and 69 years old. Males comprised 82.1% of the group

---

* Hongo 7-3-1, Bunkyo-ku, Tokyo 113, Japan (高安久雄, 小磯謙吉).

studied. Males averaged 57.4 years of age, while the mean age of females was 55 years.

3. Histological classification of bladder tumors

Primary bladder tumors were divided into 2 groups; epithelial and nonepithelial; there were 123 patients with an epithelial tumor. According to the classification of the main cells constituting the tumors, 3 types of epithelial bladder tumors occurred: Transitional, squamous, and undifferentiated. In addition, there were adenomatous tumors which arose mainly from the urachal duct. Adenomatous tumors from the bladder mucosa were rare (6).

Histological distribution of the bladder tumors in 123 patients were as follows:

Transitional cell carcinoma	113 cases (91.9%)
Adenocarcinoma	6 cases (4.9%)
Squamous cell carcinoma	3 cases (2.4%)
Undifferentiated carcinoma	1 case (0.8%)

4. Extent of tumor invasion into the bladder wall

During the 1960s these cases were staged first according to Marshall's classification (10), based on the penetration of the bladder wall. Later, Marshall's staging was demonstrated to be compatible with the T classification by UICC (18). Therefore, they were reclassified by the T classification. Classification of 113 cases of transitional cell carcinoma was as follows: T_{IS}: 0 cases (0%), T_1: 59 cases (52.2%), T_2: 31 cases (27.4%), T_3: 15 cases (13.3%), T_4: 8 cases (7.1%).

5. Grade of malignancy

The grade of malignancy was determined mainly according to Broders (21). Analysis of 113 cases of transitional cell carcinoma was as follows: Grade I: 36 cases (31.9%), Grade II: 50 cases (44.2%), Grade III: 18 cases (15.9%), Grade IV: 9 cases (8.0%).

6. Diagnosis of the bladder tumor

Cystoscopy: The first step in diagnosis is to demonstrate tumors in the bladder by cystoscopy. However, in the case of infiltrating and in situ carcinoma, it was not always easy to make a correct diagnosis. By cystoscopic procedures, the size, surface, extent of invasion, location, and shape of tumors should be observed carefully. Observation of both ureteral orifices was made carefully to examine upper urinary tract invasion.

Cystoscopic analysis of 123 cases is presented; there were 85 solitary cases (69.1%) and 38 multiple cases (30.9%), which were in good agreement with those previously reported (14).

The location of solitary tumors was classified according to Mostofi. Forty-eight point two percent of the tumors were found on the lateral walls, 20.2% on the posterior wall, 17.6% on the trigone, 7% on the vertex, 3.5% on the anterior wall, and 3.5% spread over the bladder walls.

Cystoscopic findings as to the shape of the bladder tumors were analyzed according to Melicow (12). Papillary tumors were found in 67.5%, while nonpapillary tumors were found in 32.5%.

Biopsy specimens (21) and diagnosis: The purpose of the biopsy is to make a correct diagnosis of bladder tumors by determination of tumor type, cellular type, grade, and extent of invasion. Under spinal anesthesia, biopsies were usually performed by transurethral resection which included the tumor with a portion of the bladder wall. After the establishment of diagnosis, determination of the extent of tumor invasion was made.

In addition to these procedures, the following examinations are also made: 1) Physical examination (bimanual examination of the tumor under anesthesia). 2) Roentgenograms of the chest and pelvis. 3) Plain films of kidneys, ureters, and bladder. Intravenous pyelography. 4) Urinalysis and complete blood cell count. 5) Lymphangiography and pelvic angiography, used as indicated. 6) Cystograms taken in various directions (20).

Results of the Treatment of Bladder Tumors in the University of Tokyo Hospital

In the treatment of bladder tumors, the shape, the location, number, size, and grade should be taken into account. The extent of invasion was the supreme factor in the treatment (20). However, other factors should not be ignored. There are three main methods of treatment: Surgery, radiation, and chemotherapy. In the present paper analysis of the patients who underwent surgical therapy was made. The results were expressed as relative 5-year survival rates ($\pm 2\sigma r$) (8).

1. Surgical treatment of bladder cancer (Table I)

Transurethral electroresection and coagulation (TUR, TUC): T_1 bladder tumors could be treated by TUC. However, in a case of papillary carcinoma with a broad base, TUR was the choice of therapy. Though not used in all cases, TUR and TUC were generally used on T_1 and T_2 bladder tumors. The relative 5-year survival rate of 54 patients with transitional cell carcinoma was 0.887 ± 0.116. Concerning the degree of invasion, 51 of 54 patients had a superficial lesion, T_1 and T_2, the remainder had T_3 and T_4. Two patients with T_3 bladder tumors had mutiple papillary tumors, while one patient had a T_4 solitary solid tumor. TUR and TUC were done on these 3 patients for obtaining specimens and therapy. From the clinical pictures it was assumed that total cystectomy was indicated; however, they refused such a major operation.

Grading analysis of 54 patients was demonstrated as follows: Grade I: 31 cases, Grade II: 21 cases, Grade III: 0 case, Grade IV: 2 cases. The Grade IV patients showed a poor prognosis, one survived for 2 months and the other for 3 years.

TABLE I. Results of Various Treatment for Patients with Bladder Tumor
(Relative Survival Rate $\pm 2\sigma r$)

Year	TUC, TUR	Sectio alta electrofulguration	Partial cystectomy	Total cystectomy
1	0.974 ± 0.053	0.820 ± 0.082	0.791 ± 0.248	0.674 ± 0.330
2	0.967 ± 0.064	0.793 ± 0.244	0.749 ± 0.282	0.569 ± 0.412
3	0.981 ± 0.063	0.760 ± 0.370	0.642 ± 0.359	0.577 ± 0.406
4	0.937 ± 0.092	0.786 ± 0.261	0.656 ± 0.351	0.586 ± 0.400
5	0.887 ± 0.116	0.747 ± 0.293	0.571 ± 0.420	0.450 ± 0.518
	$(n=54)$	$(n=20)$	$(n=18)$	$(n=18)$

Sectio alta with electroresection and coagulation: This operation was used for cases in which TUR and TUC were difficult to perform due to the location and number of the tumors, even though the lesion was superficial. The indication was the same as for TUR and TUC. In some cases radon-seed implantation was done. (At present this is not in clinical use.) The relative 5-year survival rate in 20 cases of transitional cell carcinoma was 0.747 ± 0.293. All the 6 patients with T_1 bladder tumors survived for 5 years after the operation. Of 10 patients with T_2 bladder tumors 4 died within 5 years. Of 3 patients with T_3 and 1 with T_4 bladder tumors all died within 5 years. These patients could not undergo the radical operation because of poor surgical risk.

A Grade I patient survived for more than 5 years, while 4 of 12 Grade II patients died within 5 years. Two of 4 Grade III patients and 1 of 3 Grade IV patients survived for more than 5 years.

Partial cystectomy: Partial cystectomy was performed on the localised and infiltrating tumors which could not be treated by transurethral and sectio alta operation. Tumors arising from the trigone could also be treated by this operation with ureteroneocystostomy. The relative 5-year survival rate in 18 partially cystectomised patients with transitional cell carcinoma was 0.571 ± 0.420. Owing to invasiveness, 5 of 6 patients with T_1, 2 of 5 patients with T_2, 2 of 6 patients with T_3, and no patient with T_4, survived more than 5 years. Concerning the grade, both Grade I patients, 5 of 8 Grade II patients, 2 of 7 Grade III patients, and no Grade IV patients survived for more than 5 years.

Total cystectomy: Total cystectomy aims at the complete removal of bladder tumors and a permanent cure. However, it was necessary to perform a urinary diversion operation, so that the surgical risk became severe.

In this hospital 14 patients with transitional cell carcinoma were operated upon by simple total cystectomy and four radical cystectomies. The relative 5-year survival rate was 0.450 ± 0.518. Concerning the invasion, 1 of 4 patients with T_1, 4 of 8 patients with T_2, 1 of 4 patients with T_3, and neither of 2 patients with T_4, survived for more than 5 years. All the patients with T_1 showed multiple papillary carcinoma which was considered not to be treated by other procedures. Concerning the grades, 1 of 3 Grade I patients, 4 of 7 Grade II patients, 1 of 6 Grade III patients, and no Grade IV, survived for more than 5 years.

The five-year survival rates with the means of urinary diversion was as follows: Ureterocutaneostomy (10 cases), 30.0%; ileal conduit (5 cases), 20.0%; ureterosigmoidostomy (3 cases), 67.0%. There were 3 patients with transitional cell carcinoma who could not undergo operation due to poor surgical risk among other reasons.

Five-year survival rates other than transitional cell carcinoma: Adenocarcinoma (6 cases), 0.409; squamous cell carcinoma (3 cases), 0.330; undifferentiated (1 case), 0.

Recurrences: Recurrences were one of the factors which influenced the prognosis. The rates of recurrence in each operative procedure were as follows: TUR, TUC: 53.7%, sectio alta with electroresection and coagulation: 47.4%, partial cystectomy: 70.0%, total cystectomy: 33.8% (local pelvic recurrences).

2. Radiation and chemotherapy (21)

Bladder tumor patients were treated mainly by operative procedures. Radiation and chemotherapy were used as adjuvant therapies. External radiation and radon-seed implantation were performed in this hospital. Local or systemic use of chemotherapeutic agents, such as mitomycin C and 5-fluorouracil, was adopted. However, there were a few cases who received these procedures, so that a complete evaluation could not be obtained.

DISCUSSION AND REVIEW

There are many methods of treatment for bladder tumor. Before the determination of therapy, the patients' occupation, habits, and mental disposition to this malignancy should be taken into account. In addition to these circumstances, the nature and extent of bladder cancer should be considered. The principles of treatment used in this hospital are as follows: Generally, transurethral electroresection and coagulation were performed on the superficial accessible lesion, while suprapubic resection (sectio alta) with fulguration was done on less accessible superficial lesions. Segmental resection was the operation of choice for the deeply infiltrating lsions located at a distance from the bladder neck. Total cystectomy with urinary diversion was performed on the patients who could not be controlled by the methods stated above (5). In some cases, adjuvant therapies, such as chemotherapy and irradiation therapy, were employed if indicated.

The relative 5-year survival rates with T_1 and T_2 bladder patients treated by TUC and/or TUR were reported as shown in Table II.

TABLE II. Results of the Relative 5-Year Survival Rates with T_1 and T_2 Bladder Patients Treated Endoscopicallly

Reporters	Invasion, T_1 (%)	Invasion, T_2 (%)
Milner (13)	70	57
Flocks (4)	77	47
Nichols and Marshall (15)	84	20
Barnes et al. (1)	63	40
Takayasu and Koiso	89.6	80.9

In our study series they were 89.6% for T_1 and 80.9% for T_2, which were good results, better results than other reporters. However, it was shown that the recurrence rate by TUC and TUR was 53.7% in this hospital, while those of Riches (17) and Pyrah (16) were 73 and 70%, respectively. From these facts, it was assumed that there were many patients who underwent TUC or TUR several times.

The relative 5-year survival rates by transvesical electroresection and coagulation were reported to be 66% by Riches (17) and 87.5% by Yoshida (22). In our study series it was 74.7%. Recurrence after this mode of therapy was 47.4%, which corresponded well with that of TUC and TUR. Essentially there were no great differences between endoscopic procedures and transvesical surgery, so that the recurrence rate between the 2 groups did not differ greatly.

Partial cystectomy has been controversial as a treatment of bladder cancer. Reports of the results of segmental cystectomy ranged from satisfactory to most unsatisfactory. Concerning 5-year survival rates Marshall (11) reported 45.2%, Jewett (7) 28.2%, and Cox (3) 41.7%. In this country Ichikawa (6) reported 45%, Yoshida

(22) 68.3%, and Suzuki (19) 75%. In our hospital it was 57.1%. Though a fair prognosis was obtained in superficial lesion, the prognosis was poor in T_3 and T_4 bladder tumors. Long (9) reported that in T_3 and T_4 patients the 5-year survival rate was between 11 and 23% after segmental cystectomy. In our study series a poorer prognosis was obtained in T_3 and T_4. Though segmental cystectomy had advantages over total cystectomy, keeping the vesical and sexual function, the recurrence rate was high. It was 70% in our results. Resection of the tumor with at least a 2-cm margin of the healthy surrounding tissues was usually performed in this clinic.

Total cystectomy was usually performed upon the deeply infiltrating bladder tumors, but superficial lesions with special reference to the number, size, location, and shape, should be the choice of operation. There are 2 types of total cystectomy: Simple and radical. Bowles and Cordonnier (2) recommended that simple cystectomy should be the operation of choice in the case of a superficial lesion, because many surgical risks exist when radical cystectomy with urinary diversion is performed. In this clinic this principle was adopted in most cases of total cystectomy. The relative 5-year survival rate in totally cystectomized patients was 0.450.

Ichikawa (6) reported the 5-year survival rate as 26% and Yoshida (22) 30.8%. Compared with the reports the results obtained were fairly good. One of the reasons for these good results was thought to be that 12 of the 18 patients belonged to T_1 and T_2. However, this was mainly due to strict indication, patient selection, and post-operative care.

Ichikawa (6) and Yoshida (22) reported on urinary diversion that ileal conduit formation was much better than ureterosigmoidostomy and ureterocutaneostomy in terms of 5-year survival. In the present study series, however, it was 67.0% in uretero-sigmoidostomy. There were a few cases of adenocarcinoma, squamous cell carcinoma, and undifferentiated carcinoma, so that a complete evaluation could not be obtained.

REFERENCES

1. Barnes, R. W., Bergman, R. T., Hadley, H. L., and Love, D. Control of bladder tumors by endoscopic surgery. *J. Urol.*, **97**, 864–868 (1967).
2. Bowles, W. T. and Cordonnier, J. J. Total cystectomy for carcinoma of the bladder. *J. Urol.*, **90**, 731–735 (1963).
3. Cox, C. E., Cass, A. S., and Boyce, W. H. Bladder cancer; A 26-year review. *J. Urol.*, **101**, 550–558 (1969).
4. Flocks, R. H. Treatment of carcinoma of bladder. *J. Am. Med. Assoc.*, **145**, 295–300 (1951).
5. Henry, W. F. and Bloom, H.J.G. Urothelial neoplasma; Present position and prospects. *Recent Adv. Urol.*, **2**, 245–292 (1976).
6. Ichikawa, T. Remote results of bladder tumors. *Nippon Hinyokika Gakkai Zasshi (Japan. J. Urol.)*, **45**, 221–224 (1954) (in Japanese).
7. Jewett, H. J., King, L. R., and Shelley, W. M. A study of 365 cases of characteristics to prognosis after extirpation. *J. Urol.*, **92**, 668–678 (1964).
8. Kurihara, N. and Takano, A. Computing method to the relative survival rates. *Gan-no-Rinsho (Cancer Clinic)*, **11**, 628–632 (1965) (in Japanese).
9. Long, R.T.L., Grummon, R. A., Spratt, J. S., and Perez-Mesa, C. Carcinoma of the

urinary bladder. (Comparison with radical, simple and partial cystectomy and intravesical formalin.) *Cancer*, **29**, 98–105 (1972).

10. Marshall, V. F. The relation of preoperative estimate to the pathogenic demonstration of the vesical neoplasma. *J. Urol.*, **68**, 714–723 (1952).

11. Marshall, V. F., Holden, J., and Ma, K. T. Survival of patients with bladder carcinoma treated by simple segmental resection. *Cancer*, **9**, 26–29 (1956).

12. Melicow, M. M. Tumors of the urinary bladder; A clinico-pathological analysis of over 2500 specimens and biopsies. *J. Urol.*, **74**, 498–521 (1955).

13. Milner, W. A. The role of conservative surgery in the treatment of bladder tumors. *Br. J. Urol.*, **26**, 375–384 (1954).

14. Mostofi, E. K. A study of 2,678 patients with initial carcinoma of the bladder. I. Survival rates. *J. Urol.*, **75**, 480–491 (1956).

15. Nichols, J. A. and Marshall, V. F. The treatment of bladder carcinoma by local excision and fulguration. *Cancer*, **9**, 559–565 (1956).

16. Pyrah, L. N, Raper, F. P., and Thomas, G. M. Report of a follow-up of papillary tumors of the bladder. *Br. J. Urol.*, **36**, 14–25 (1964).

17. Riches, S. E. Surgery and radiotherapy in urology; the bladder. *J. Urol.*, **90**, 339–350 (1963).

18. Rubin, F. Cancer of the urogenital tract; bladder cancer. *J. Am. Med. Assoc.*, **18**, 1761–1763 (1968).

19. Suzuki, K., Sugita, A., Miura, T., Kato, M., Onodera, Y., Yabuki, H., and Kato, T. Clinical and pathological studies on partial cystectomy for urinary bladder cancer. I. Clinical pictures and follow-up studies. *Nippon Hinyokika Gakkai Zasshi (Japan. J. Urol.)*, **57**, 380–387 (1966) (in Japanese).

20. Takayasu, H. and Nishiura, T. Study on ths cystogram: The first report. Aspects of the cystogram obtained in various positions with special reference to a method for roentgenological visualization of the base of the bladder. *Nippon Hinyokika Gakkai Zasshi (Japan. J. Urol.)*, **44**, 123–129 (1953) (in Japanese).

21. Takayasu, H. and Yonase, Y. Bladder cancer. *In* "Recent Surgery Series. 41B. Urology. II," Nakayama Shoten, Tokyo, pp. 84–109 (1970) (in Japanese).

22. Yoshida, O. Studies on carcinoma of the urinary bladder. *Hinyokika Kiyo (Kyoto)*, **12**, 1261–1280 (1967) (in Japanese).

GANN Monograph on Cancer Research 22, 1979

CANCER OF THE PROSTATE

Hisao Takayasu and Kenkichi Koiso

Department of Urology, Faculty of Medicine, University of Tokyo*

Results of treatment in 78 patients with prostatic carcinoma, who visited the University of Tokyo Hospital, are reviewed. The principle of treatment was anti-androgenic, using the synthetic estrogens (mainly hexestrol and diethylstilbestrol diphosphate).

The relative overall 5-year survival rate was $0.408 \pm 0.131 (2\sigma r)$. Patients without metastasis at the first visit had a relative 5-year survival rate of 0.522 ± 0.192, while those with metastasis had 0.323 ± 0.175. Forty-nine cases of well-differentiated adenocarcinoma, 25 cases of the anaplastic type and 4 unknown cases were found. Relative 5-year survival rates for the well-differentiated and the anaplastic types were 0.601 ± 0.175 and 0.098 ± 0.138, respectively. The extent of tumor invasion of prostatic carcinoma was graded according to the TNM classification. The relative 5-year survival rates for T_3 (45 cases) and $T_{3-4}NxM0$ (35 cases) were 0.462 ± 0.177 and 0.456 ± 0.201, respectively. Additionally, the relative 5-year survival rates for T_4 (26 cases) and $T_{0-4}NxM1$ (38 cases) were 0.284 ± 0.203 and 0.291 ± 0.169, respectively.

Side-effects were routinely checked and treated properly. Pathogenesis of cardiovascular accidents during estrogen therapy, which were pointed out by the Veterans' Administration Co-operative Urological Research Group, should be investigated and clarified in the future. The endocrine therapy of prostatic carcinoma has some limitations which should be overcome in the near future.

Although the morbidity of prostatic carcinoma in Japan has recently been increasing, it is still much lower than in other countries. The highest incidence of prostatic carcinoma in this country is said to be around 70 years of age and more than half of all cases are at T_3 when first seen (*12*).

As with benign prostatic hypertrophy, there are many problems to be solved as far as the treatment of prostatic carcinoma is concerned. In 1941, Huggins demonstrated that estrogen administration had a dramatic effect on the treatment of prostatic carcinoma (*10*). Since then, anti-androgenic therapy has been widely accepted and used in Japan. Synthetic estrogen preparations have been administered, routinely combined with castration. Sometimes progressively higher doses of estrogen preparations were given. However, the efficiency of hormone management has been seriously questioned by recent investigations of the Veterans' Administration Co-operative Urological Research Group, because of the high incidence of cardiovascular accidents brought by estrogen administration (*17, 18*).

---

* Hongo 7-3-1, Bunkyo-ku, Tokoy 113, Japan (高安久雄, 小磯謙吉).

This paper presents a review and the results of treatment of prostatic carcinoma, during 1963–1969, in the University of Tokyo Hospital.

Principles of Diagnosis and Treatment

From 1963 to 1969, 78 patients visited our hospital. The average age was 67.8 years; the range was 45 to 86 years. Of these patients 80.8% were between 60 and 79 years. All the patients who visited our hospital received the anti-androgenic therapy.

Diagnosis of prostatic carcinoma was chiefly made by prostatic biopsy. (Needle biopsies were mainly employed, but sometimes aspiration biopsies were made.) The transurethral, transrectal, and transperineal routes were chosen. Biopsy specimens were sent to the Department of Pathology for pathological diagnosis. After the diagnosis was established, determination of the extent of the disease should be made.

Preliminary studies included the following:

1) Physical examination (rectal palpation of the prostate).
2) Roentgenograms of the chest, lumbar portion of the supine and pelvis.
3) Plain films of the kidneys, ureters, and bladder. Intravenous pyelography.
4) Urinalysis and complete blood count (CBC).
5) Determination of the serum levels of acid and alkaline phosphatases.
6) Cystoscopy and urethroscopy (Sigmoidoscopy was seldom indicated.).
7) Bone marrow biopsies or bone marrow aspiration.
8) Radioactive bone scanning of the pelvis and lumbar portion.
9) Lymphangiography.

Radioactive bone scanning and lymphangiography were performed towards the end of the 1960s.

From these studies the grading and extent of invasion of the prostatic carcinoma were determined. Even though there were some disputes concerning the determination and classification of staging, the TNM classification according to UICC was adopted in this paper (*9*).

As prostatic carcinoma is a malignant disease, radical resection of the prostate (total prostatectomy) is the treatment of choice. However, when first seen, a very low percentage of the prostatic cancer patients were candidates for radical operation in clinical practice. Two patients, one with T_1 and the other with T_2, were aged over 70 years, so that no patients deserved radical operation. Therefore, anti-androgenic treatment was mainly employed in our hospital. It is said that in the treatment of prostatic carcinoma estrogens act as the hormone suppressing the axis of hypothalamus-hypophysis-adrenals-gonads, so that adrenal and gonadal androgenic activities are lowered. This principle is based on the fact that the growth and metabolism of the prostatic epithelial cells are influenced and controlled by the androgenic hormone, especially testosterone, produced and secreted from the adrenals and testes. Other investigators have stated that estrogens are potent anticancer agents, which directly act upon the prostatic cancer cells (*4*). On this principle, relatively large doses of synthetic estrogens were administered. Hexestrol and diethylstilbestrol diphosphate were the drugs of choice. Castration was also performed in almost every case.

Efficiency of the treatment was estimated by the signs and symptoms, and the results were expressed as the relative 5-year survival rate. In addition, pathological examination of the prostatic cancer cells was usually made with Hematoxylin-Eosin staining. Most of the prostatic carcinomas were adenocarcinomas.

Anti-androgenic Treatment in the University of Tokyo Hospital

Of 78 patients, 80.8% were between 60 and 79 years old. The tumor was rare below the age of 50 (1.3%), and after the age of 80 clinical cases were less common (7.7%). Chief complaints were dysuria, urinary retention, hematuria, lumbago, frequency, and neuralgia, which were in accordance with those of benign prostatic hypertrophy, except the neuralgia.

Pathological examination of prostatic specimens, taken by needle biopsy or other methods, revealed the following:

Well-differentiated adenocarcinoma	49 cases
Anaplastic type of prostatic carcinoma	25 cases
Unknown	4 cases

Adenocarcinoma of the prostate predominated in this study. The relative overall 5-year survival rate of prostatic carcinoma in our hospital was estimated as 0.408 ± 0.131 (Table I).

The relative 5-year survival rate was compared between well-differentiated adenocarcinoma and the anaplastic type of prostatic carcinoma. It was 0.601 ± 0.175 in the former and 0.098 ± 0.138 in the latter; there was a great difference between the two groups. Prognosis of the anaplastic type was much worse than that of the well-differentiated type (Table II).

Grading of prostatic carcinoma was also made. However, in clinical practice it was enough to grade into two categories; low and high grade. Well-differentiated tumors had a low-grade character and anaplastic type tumors had a high grade. It was also assumed that the higher the grade, the poorer the prognosis.

The extent of the primary tumor invasion of 78 patients with prostatic carcinoma was described by TNM classification. The results were as follows:

TABLE I.   Results of Treatment for Patients with Prostatic Carcinoma

Years	Overall relative survival rate $(\pm 2\sigma r)$
1	0.825 ± 0.111
2	0.721 ± 0.148
3	0.580 ± 0.195
4	0.488 ± 0.228
5	0.408 ± 0.131

TABLE II.   Relative Survival Rates $(\pm 2\sigma r)$ in Patients with the Well-differentiated and Anaplastic Types of Prostatic Carcinoma

Years	Well-differentiated	Anaplastic
1	0.868 ± 0.095	0.788 ± 0.177
2	0.862 ± 0.124	0.562 ± 0.216
3	0.740 ± 0.154	0.362 ± 0.211
4	0.680 ± 0.168	0.190 ± 0.178
5	0.601 ± 0.175	0.098 ± 0.138

1) T classification
T_0 5 cases (6.4%)
T_1 1 case (1.3%)
T_2 1 case (1.3%)
T_3 45 cases (57.7%)
T_4 26 cases (33.3%)

2) TNM classification
T_0NxM_0 4 cases (5.1%)
$T_{1-2}NxM_0$ 1 case (1.3%)
$T_{3-4}NxM_0$ 35 cases (44.9%)
$T_{0-4}NxM_1$ 38 cases (48.7%)

As already pointed out, there were fewer patients in the low grade of prostatic carcinoma. The relative 5-year survival rates in each group are shown in Tables III, IV, and V. Five patients with T_0 survived for 5 years.

Results of treatment by estrogen preparations should be evaluated in the patients with or without metastasis when first seen. The relative 5-year survival rate of the nonmetastatic group was 0.522 ± 0.192, while it was 0.323 ± 0.175 in the metastatic group. Metastasis was one of the poor prognostic signs in this malignancy. It was usually found in the pelvic bones, vertebrae, and ribs as an osteoblastic lesion. Metastases were found in 48.7% of the observed patients when first seen.

TABLE III. Relative Survival Rate ($\pm 2\sigma r$) in T_3 and T_4 Patients with Prostatic Carcinoma

Years	T_3	T_4
1	0.853 ± 0.134	0.758 ± 0.180
2	0.745 ± 0.185	0.634 ± 0.210
3	0.603 ± 0.247	0.479 ± 0.219
4	0.502 ± 0.175	0.366 ± 0.215
5	0.462 ± 0.177	0.284 ± 0.203

TABLE IV. Relative Survival Rate ($\pm 2\sigma r$) in $T_{3-4}NxM0$ and $T_{0-4}NxM1$ Patients with Prostatic Carcinoma

Years	$T_{3-4}NxM0$	$T_{1-4}NxM1$
1	0.889 ± 0.123	0.738 ± 0.153
2	0.772 ± 0.165	0.626 ± 0.173
3	0.646 ± 0.167	0.447 ± 0.179
4	0.543 ± 0.200	0.345 ± 0.175
5	0.456 ± 0.201	0.291 ± 0.169

TABLE V. Relative Survival Rate ($\pm 2\sigma r$) in Patients with Prostatic Carcinoma with or without Metastasis at the first Visit

Years	Without metastasis	With metastasis
1	0.908 ± 0.146	0.778 ± 0.142
2	0.811 ± 0.148	0.654 ± 0.171
3	0.707 ± 0.173	0.474 ± 0.181
4	0.624 ± 0.188	0.376 ± 0.179
5	0.522 ± 0.192	0.323 ± 0.175

TABLE VI. Results of Treatments on Patients with Prostatic Carcinoma Given Hexestrol at a Daily Dose of 30 or 100 mg; Relative Survival Rate ($\pm 2\sigma r$)

Years	30-mg group	100-mg group
1	0.785 ± 0.146	0.778 ± 0.142
2	0.643 ± 0.174	0.716 ± 0.162
3	0.490 ± 0.184	0.600 ± 0.176
4	0.419 ± 0.132	0.499 ± 0.153
5	0.294 ± 0.172	0.462 ± 0.188

Serum phosphatases, acid and alkaline, were said to be one of the reliable parameters in estimating and diagnosing the course of prostatic carcinoma. Levels of serum acid phosphatase were determined in 77 patients, at the first visit to this hospital, by Bessey's method. Thirty-three patients were within the normal limits, while it was elevated in 44 patients. Relative 5-year survival rates for the 2 groups were 0.479 ± 0.208 and 0.362 ± 0.169, respectively.

Serum alkaline phosphatases were determined in 77 patients. It was elevated in 35 patients. Relative 5-year survival rates for the elevated and nonelevated groups were 0.351 ± 0.188 in the elevated, and 0.464 ± 0.184 in the normal group, respectively.

According to Furgusson (8) a relatively high-dose therapy (hexestrol 100 mg/day) was employed in 40 cases, while in 37 patients a 30 mg/day dose of hexestrol was given. Relative 5-year survival rates in the 100-mg and 30-mg dose groups were 0.462 ± 0.188 and 0.294 ± 0.172, respectively (Table VI).

In the course of estrogen therapy, several complications were found, such as gynecomastia, edema, hypertension and liver dysfunction. They were treated appropriately.

When prostatic carcinoma invaded and obstructed the urinary tracts, release of the obstruction by transurethral resection of the prostatic tumor, cystostomy, ureterostomy, and indwelling of the balloon catheter were performed. Of 78 patients at the first visit such procedures were required in 26.

DISCUSSION AND REVIEW

Prostatic carcinoma is often asymptomatic. There are no great differences in symptoms between benign prostatic hypertrophy and prostatic malignancy, except neuralgia. The most common symptoms associated with prostatic carcinoma were either obstruction or neuralgia. According to Chisholm (4) prostatic carcinoma in some cases manifests its existence as bone metastasis: Occult cancer of the prostate and latent carcinoma of the prostate are found at prostatectomy or autopsy. In the present study series, no occult carcinoma was found, while latent carcinoma was demonstrated in 5 cases.

According to Bumpus (2) the average age at onset of prostatic carcinoma was 65 with half occurring between 60 and 70 years. In our series most of the patients were aged between 60 and 79, which agreed with the literature.

There are many methods of treatment for prostatic carcinoma (11). Endocrine therapy with castration was chosen as a main therapeutic principle. Historically, the treatment of prostatic carcinoma only included relieving urinary obstruction and pain before the discovery of hormone therapy. Radiation therapy was adopted but soon abandoned. In 1941, Huggins and Hodges published the first successful results of treating this malignancy by estrogens (*10*). Since then there have been many reports on the results of estrogen treatment (*1, 7, 14, 15*). To summarize these reports, there is little doubt that castration and/or estrogen treatment influences the shrinkage of prostatic tumor, decreasing the levels of serum acid phosphatase and control of metastasis. In addition to this, the patients may have a striking subjective improvement. Our data of relative overall 5-year survival rate was 0.408, for those patients without metastasis 0.522, for those with metastasis 0.323. In 1960 Emmett et al. (*6*) reviewed the results of their hormone therapy; the 5-year survival rate was fairly good. They recommended that early orchiectomy with estrogen therapy should be used for prostatic cancer therapy.

A major problem in endocrine treatment has been the unpredictable course of this malignancy. It appeared that failure to respond to anti-androgenic therapy was more probable in an undifferentiated carcinoma. In our study, there was a great difference in the relative 5-year survival rates between the well-differentiated and the anaplastic types. It was assumed that susceptability to the endocrine hormone differed between the two types.

On the basis that estrogens act as a chemotherapeutic agent, large doses of estrogen (100 mg of hexestrol daily) were given to 40 patients (*13*). Clinical data from this study indicated that when hexestrol was used, there seemed to be some difference in relative 5-year survival rates between the 100-mg and 30-mg dose groups, consisting of 40 and 37 cases, respectively, as Furgusson recommended a high dose of stilbestrol therapy.

There are many estrogen preparations which were used to suppress the androgenic function. In Japan diethylstilbestrol diphosphate and hexestrol have been widely used. Other estrogens, natural or synthetic, and synthetic progesterones also were in clinical use. There was a tendency to show lack of responsiveness to the endocrine therapy during the treatment. The precise mechanism of this phenomenon has yet to be elucidated. In such cases cytotoxic drugs and anticancer antibiotics were used.

External radiation therapy has been abandoned because of inefficacy. With the introduction of supervoltage irradiation it has been employed at several hospitals in this country. Tsuya et al. (*16*) summarized the recent results of stage C prostatic carcinoma. The 5-year survival rate was 40%, which was in good agreement with those of Regato and Carlton (*3, 5*).

Side-effects of estrogens should be checked periodically and managed appropriately. Recently, the Veterans' Administration Co-operative Urological Research Group criticized the estrogen treatment of prostatic carcinoma, analyzing the larger scale results: Study I, II, and III (*17, 18*). They concluded that cardiovascular hazards of estrogens were noted during estrogen therapy and, owing to these facts, estrogen therapy not only failed to increase the length of survival, but also there was a higher incidence of cardiovascular death. There have been several criticisms of these trials. In our autopsied cases there were no cardiovascular deaths which were clearly demonstrated to be due to estrogen therapy. However, pathogenesis of cardiovascular accidents during estrogen therapy, pointed out by the Veterans' Administration Co-operative Urological Research Group, should be investigated and clarified in the future.

REFERENCES

1. Barnes, R. W. and Ninan, C. A. Carcinoma of the prostate. Biopsy and conservative therapy. *J. Urol.*, **108**, 897–900 (1972).
2. Bumpus, H. C. Carcinoma of the prostate; a clinical study of 100 cases. *Surg. Gynecol. Obstet.*, **43**, 150–155 (1926).
3. Carlton, C. E., Jr., Dawould, F., Hudgins, P., and Scott, R., Jr. Irradiation treatment of the prostate; a preliminary report based on 8 years of experience. *J. Urol.*, **108**, 924–927 (1972).
4. Chisholm, G. D. Conservative treatment of cancer of the prostate. *In* "The Treatment of Prostatic Hypertrophy and Neoplasia," ed. by J. E. Castro, Medical and Technical Publishing Co. Ltd., Lancaster, pp. 121–130 (1974).
5. Del Regato, J. A. Radiotherapy in conservative treatment of operable and locally inoperable carcinoma of the prostate. *Radiology*, **88**, 761–766 (1967).
6. Emmett, J. L., Greene, L. F., and Papantoniou, A. Endocrine therapy in carcinoma of the prostate gland: 10-year survival studies. *J. Urol.*, **83**, 471–484 (1960).
7. Farnsworth, W. E. A direct effect of estrogens on prostatic metabolism of testosterone. *J. Invest. Urol.*, **6**, 423–427 (1969).
8. Fergusson, J. D. Carcinoma of the prostate. *Trans. Med. Soc. (London)*, **83**, 92–95 (1967).
9. Gardner, W. V. Report on the TNM classification. Proposal for Bladder, Prostate, Kidney, Testis. International Union Against Cancer, Geneva (1968).
10. Huggins, C. and Hodges, C. V. Studies on prostatic cancer: 1. The effect of castration, of estrogen, and of androgen injection on serum phosphatases in metastatic carcinoma of the prostate. *Cancer Res.*, **1**, 1317–1320 (1950).
11. Nesbit, R. M. and Baum, W. C. Endocrine control of prostatic carcinoma: Clinical and statistical survey of 1818 cases. *J. Am. Med. Assoc.*, **143**, 1317–1320 (1950).
12. Okada, K. Prostatic carcinoma in Japanese. *Rinsho Hinyokika (Clinical Urology, Tokyo)*, **27**, 765–769 (1973) (in Japanese).
13. Robinson, M.R.G. and Thomas, B. C. Effect of hormonal therapy on plasma testosterone levels in prostatic carcinoma. *Br. Med. J.*, **4**, 391–394 (1971).
14. Rubin, D. Cancer of the urogenital tract prostatic cancer. *J. Am. Med. Assoc.*, **210**, 322–323 (1969).
15. Segal, S. J., Marberger, H., and Flocks, R. H. Tissue distribution of stilbestrol diphosphates; concentration in prostatic tissue. *J. Urol.*, **81**, 474–478 (1959).
16. Tsuya, A., Kawai, T., Fukushima, S., Shida, K., Shimazaki, J., Matsumoto, K., and Seto, T. Radiotherapy combined with hormone therapy for prostatic cancer. *Strahlentherapie*, **148**, 24–34 (1974).
17. The Veterans' Administration Co-operative Urological Research Group. Treatment and survival of patients with cancer of the prostate. *Surg. Gynecol. Obstet.*, **126**, 1011–1017 (1967).
18. The Veterans' Administration Co-operative Urological Research Group. Carcinoma of the prostate; treatment comparisons. *J. Urol.*, **98**, 516–522 (1967).

CANCER OF THE UTERINE CERVIX IN JAPAN

Koji HIRABAYASHI

Department of Obstetrics and Gynecology,
*Okayama University Medical School**

The Japan Uterine Cancer Committee was established in 1952. The number of hospitals co-operating with the Committee has increased from 22 in 1953 to 169 in 1978. Further, the number of treated cases listed by the Committee has increased from 4,253 cases in 1953–1954 to 13,331 cases in 1973–1974. In regard to the distribution of clinical stage, the rate of Stage I carcinoma has nearly doubled during the past 22 years and the rate of Stage II and III carcinoma has markedly decreased. Concerning the treatment results, slight but steady improvement in surgical treatment and significant improvement in radiotherapy were noted during the period of 1953–1969. However, the treatment results had not improved as much as expected when an overall examination was made of the treatment results in Japan. The cause was investigated and it was concluded that even though the screening for early detection of carcinoma must be carried out on as wide a basis as possible, its treatment should be performed on a concentric basis. Progress in the method of treatment during the period from 1953 to 1974 was reviewed. There is a characteristically high rate of surgery for treating Stages I and II but more reduced surgical methods have been applied to cases of Stage Ia carcinoma. Preoperative irradiation has not yielded any beneficial effect and postoperative irradiation is now carried out on selected cases which have a high possibility of residual carcinoma. The main source of external irradiation is ^{60}Co (60%), followed by supervoltage Linac and β-tron (39%). As to intracavitary irradiation, the afterloading system with radium, ^{60}Co, or ^{137}Cs is now in wide use in Japan.

Registration and Management of Carcinoma of the Uterine Cervix in Japan

In 1952, The Japan Uterine Cancer Committee was established within The Japan Society of Obstetrics and Gynecology to list and maintain a close check on patients with carcinoma of the cervix and of the uterine body. In the first year (1953), there were only 22 hospitals co-operating with the Committee but now there are 165 such hospitals throughout Japan. The number of cases with carcinoma of the cervix listed by the Committee from 1953 to 1954 were 4,253 and this rose during a 20-year period ot 13,331 in 1973–1974.

* Shikata 2-5-1, Okayama 700, Japan (平林光司).

Changes in Clinical Stage Distribution

Figure 1 indicates the changes which have taken place with regard to the clinical stages of the disease. The frequency of the stages was in the order of Stage II, III, I, and IV during 1953–1954 and Stage I, II, III, and IV during 1973–1974. A remarkable change was observed from 1963 to 1964 in the form of a sudden increase in Stage I and a marked decrease in Stage II and III. This was a result of the increased efficiency in the early detection of cancer attained during this period. It is pleasing to note that the rate of Stage I carcinoma has nearly doubled during the past 22 years, but this also indicates the increasing necessity for the detection of cancer in its early stages, as Stage III and IV still account for 25.8% of cases.

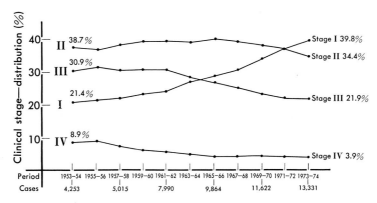

Fig. 1.   Change of clinical stage-distribution
   Significant increase in Stage I and significant decrease in Stages II, III, and IV (1953–1954: 1973–1974).

Treatment Results during 1953–1969

1.   Evaluation method for treatment results

According to the rules of The Cancer Committee of International Federation of Gynecology and Obstetrics (FIGO), the treatment results were evaluated by the observed 5-year survival rate, that is, the number of cases living after 5 years divided by the total number of treated cases. Evaluation by the relative 5-year survival rate is

TABLE I.   5-Year Results of Surgical Treatment

Period	1953–1954			1955–1957			1958–1960		
Stage	No.	5-Year survivors	%	No.	5-Year survivors	%	No.	5-Year survivors	%
I[a]	762	633	83.1	1,310	1,084	82.8	1,769	1,463	82.7
II[a]	1,165	722	62.0	1,923	1,293	67.2	2,592	1,768	68.2
III	418	186	44.5	538	263	48.9	535	261	48.4
IV	14	1	7.1	28	5	17.9	10	2	20.0
Total	2,359	1,542	65.4	3,779	2,645	69.6	4,906	3,494	71.2

[a] Significant improvement (1953–1954 : 1967–1969).

desirable but was impossible owing to the lack of birth date in the computer program of the Committee. The percentage of lost to follow-up was constantly 5.3% and death from other causes was 3.4%. Statistical analysis was made by χ^2 test (ratio or risk=5%). As will be described later, when we investigate the differences between the hospitals concerned in their abilities for treating the disease, the difference in the distribution of clinical stage should be corrected. For this purpose, the treatment result ratio proposed by Kitabatake (2) was utilized.

$$\text{Treatment result ratio} = \frac{\text{5-Year survival rate}}{\text{Stage index}}$$

$$\text{Stage index} = \frac{aA + bB + cC + dD}{N} \qquad \text{where: } N = \text{total number}$$

expected survival rate
$a = 0.85,\ b = 0.65,\ c = 0.45,\ c = 0.10$

$A,\ B,\ C,\ D$—number of cases of
Stages I, II, III, and IV.

2.   Surgical treatment

The results of surgical treatment during the period of 1953–1969 are shown in Table I and Fig. 2. A significant increase in 5-year survival rate was observed in Stage I and II carcinoma.

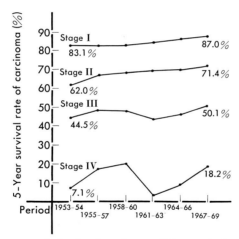

FIG. 2.   Five-year survival rate of carcinoma of the cervix (surgery)
Significant improvement was observed in Stage I and II (1953–1954: 1967–1969).

in Carcinoma of the Cervix in Japan (1953–1969)

	1961–1963			1964–1966			1967–1969		
No.	5-Year survivors	%	No.	5-Year survivors	%	No.	5-Year survivors	%
2,671	2,242	83.9	3,553	3,047	85.8	3,805	3,311	87.0
3,694	2,547	69.0	4,296	2,994	69.7	3,852	2,751	71.4
812	351	43.2	757	346	45.9	511	256	50.1
27	1	3.7	23	2	8.7	11	2	18.2
5,947	4,150	69.8	8,626	6,389	74.1	8,179	6,320	77.3

TABLE II.   Five-year Results of Radiotherapy in

Period	1953–1954			1955–1957			1958–1960		
Stage	No.	5-Year survivors	%	No.	5-Year survivors	%	No.	5-Year survivors	%
I[a]	136	75	55.2	163	113	69.3	345	226	65.5
II[a]	464	198	42.7	662	350	52.9	991	538	54.3
III[a]	916	229	24.9	1,579	442	28.0	2,282	678	29.7
IV	378	37	9.8	512	60	11.7	559	80	14.3
Total	1,894	539	28.5	2,916	965	33.1	4,177	1,522	36.4

[a] Significant improvement (1953–1954 : 1967–1969).

3.   Radiotherapy

The results of radiotherapy are shown in Table II and Fig. 3. An increase in 5-year survival rate was seen at each stage. The results shown here include those up to 1969. As will be described later, supervoltage radiotherapy was in wide use at this time. There is no doubt that there will be future improvement in the results of radiotherapy.

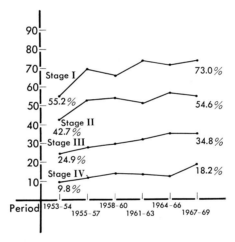

FIG. 3.   Five-year survival rate of carcinoma of the cervix (radiotherapy)
Significant improvement was observed in Stages I, II, and III (1953–1954: 1967–1969).

Investigation of the Cancer Control Activity of Hospitals

It was disappointing to find that the results of such a treatment had not improved as expected during the past 22 years when an overall examination was made of treatment results. We therefore decided to investigate the cause. We examined the differences between the hospitals concerned in their abilities to treat such patients. We believed that there would be a difference in results between those hospitals with a small number of carcinoma patients and those with a large number of such patients. However, differences in the distribution of clinical stage would constitute a further complication. It is obvious that the treatment results would be more favorable in hospitals where Stage I and II patients were in the majority, necessitating the adjust-

Carcinoma of the Cervix in Japan (1953-1969)

1961-1963			1964-1966			1967-1969		
No.	5-Year survivors	%	No.	5-Year svrvivors	%	No.	5-Year survivors	%
435	320	73.6	535	380	71.0	641	468	73.0
1,190	608	51.1	1,470	824	56.1	1,672	913	54.6
2,961	946	32.0	3,196	1,106	34.7	2,914	1,014	34.8
585	80	13.7	594	73	12.3	522	60	11.5
5,171	1,954	37.8	5,789	2,383	41.2	5,749	2,455	42.7

ment of such data. The treatment result ratio was useful for this adjustment. The relation between the treatment result ratio and the number of cases treated per year was examined. As shown in Fig. 4 (surgery) and Fig. 5 (radiotherapy), there has been an annual improvement in treatment results at all hospitals concerned, but the results from hospitals having only a few patients are still inferior to those at hospitals which handle many cancer patients. This trend has been particularly remarkable in connection with the results of radiotherapy. Figure 6 indicates, on the basis of the afore-mentioned data, the scales of the hospitals at which patients with carcinoma of the cervix have been treated. These data reveal that about 25% of cases from 1955 to 1957 were being treated at hospitals handling over 201 cases each year, but that this figure dropped to 10.7% during 1964–1966 despite an increase in the number of patients. On the other hand, the percentage of cases treated at hospitals having less than 100 cases a year rose to 64% during 1964–1966. This was an indication that an increase in the number of

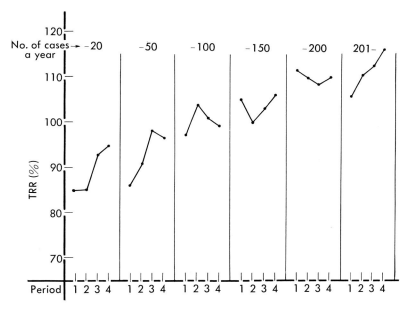

FIG. 4. Comparison of treatment result ratio (TRR) (surgery)
1, 1955–1957; 2, 1958–1960; 3, 1961–1963; 4, 1964–1966.

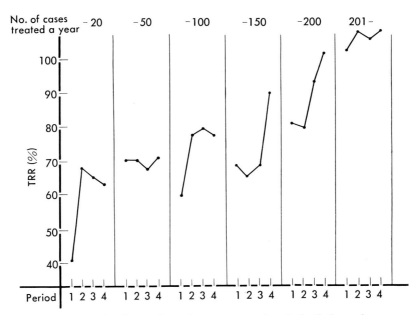

FIG. 5.   Comparison of treatment result ratio (radiotherapy)

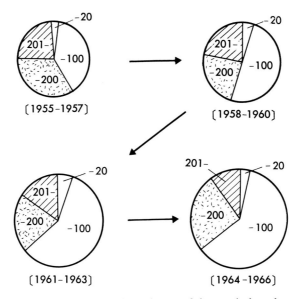

FIG. 6.   Kind of hospital in which carcinoma of the cervix have been treated in Japan
        Area of the circle is in proportion to the number of cases.

hospitals capable of coping with a small number of patients, in this case 100 or less a year, resulted in an increase in the number of patients receiving treatment. As mentioned earlier, the results of treatment at hospitals handling a small number of patients are not good. Even though there may have been an improvement in the results at individual hospitals, such an improvement overall has not been seen. This fact has an extremely important bearing on our subject as it means that even though the screening for early detection of cancer must be carried out on as wide a basis as possible, its treatment must be performed on a concentric basis.

Progress in the Method of Treatment

1. Surgical treatment
Surgical rate: As shown in Fig. 7, in Japan, a characteristically high rate of surgery in treating carcinoma of the cervix of Stage I and II has been observed. The basic operative method is Okabayashi's radical hysterectomy. In regard to the treatment of carcinoma in its early stages, surgery which constitutes a highly radical method of healing restricted carcinoma has played an important role in Japan. It also appears to have resulted in improving international results. However, radical operations are often accompanied by a variety of disturbances and they should be reduced as much as possible. However, as shown in Fig. 7, surgical treatments are gradually being performed more frequently in both Europe and America in Stage I carcinoma. It would be ideal if both sides could meet halfway and I believe this will happen in the near future.

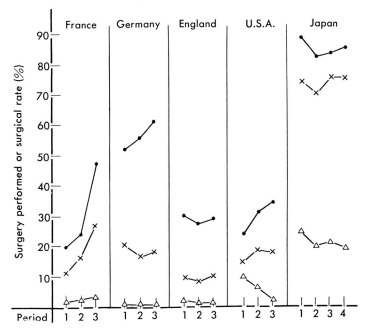

FIG. 7.   Comparison of indication of surgical treatment

Stage Ia: Recently the frequency of Stage Ia carcinoma has notably increased and more reduced operative methods have been applied to Stage Ia carcinoma. In 1974, there were 1,018 cases of Stage Ia and 662 cases (65%) were treated by modified radical, or simple hysterectomy.
Preoperative irradiation: Preoperative irradiation has been tried in several hospitals without any clear beneficial effects.

TABLE III. Application of Postoperative Irradiation

Period	No. of hospital reported	Routinely applied	No. of application	Selectively applied (%)
1953	18	17	1	0 (0.0)
1959	36	31	0	5 (13.9)
1964	97	83	3	11 (11.3)
1969	64	31	0	33 (51.6)
1974	91	32	0	59 (64.8)

Postoperative irradiation: On the other hand, as indicated in Table III, postoperative irradiation was carried out in almost all cases in 1953, however, since then such irradiation has been selectively used. The decision about the necessity for postoperative irradiation, dose, and irradiation field has been made on the basis of operative findings, radicality, and histological examination of the surgical specimen to determine how far the cancer has advanced. I would like to assert that postoperative irradiation should be carried out according to each individual.

Prophylactic vaginal cuff irradiation: Since 1957 we have been doing this radiation by placing a small radiation source at the vaginal cuff when there has been radical hysterectomy (2). There are two merits in this method; the first, shown in Fig. 8, is that there has been a remarkable decrease in recurrence at the vaginal cuff; the second is sufficient retention of the vaginal wall, thus allowing more satisfactory sexual intercourse following surgery, as a result of a longer residual vagina.

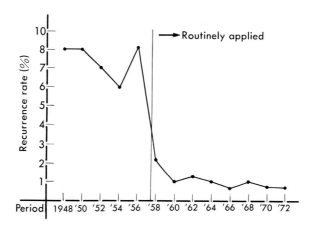

FIG. 8. Effect of prophylactic vaginal cuff irradiation method (recurrence rate at vaginal cuff)

2.   Radiotherapy

External irradiation: As shown in Table IV, instruments used for external irradiation in 1953 were all orthovoltage X-ray instruments. There has since been an increase in instruments of irradiation utilizing ^{60}Co, and these are now being used in about 60% of the hospitals concerned. Use of the supervoltage Linac and Betatron has increased since 1969, with 39% of the hospitals now utilizing it. It is certain that this supervoltage radiotherapy will be seen in even wider use in the future.

TABLE IV.   Equipment for External Irradiation

Period	No. of hospitals reported	Orthovoltage (%)	^{60}Co, ^{137}Cs (%)	Supervoltage (%)
1953	23	23 (100.0)	0 (0.0)	0 (0.0)
1959	52	35 (67.3)	16 (30.7)	1 (2.0)
1964	67	17 (25.4)	49 (73.1)	1 (1.5)
1969	63	4 (6.3)	49 (77.8)	10 (15.9)
1974	110	1 (0.9)	66 (60.0)	43 (39.1)

TABLE V.   Main Source of Intracavitary Irradiation

Period	No. of hospital reported	Radium (%)	^{60}Co (%)	^{137}Cs (%)
1953	23	23 (100.0)	0	0
1959	46	44 (95.6)	2 (4.4)	0
1964	65	54 (83.1)	11 (16.9)	0
1969	62	45 (72.6)	14 (22.6)	3 (4.8)
1974	95	53 (55.8)	30 (31.6)	12 (12.6)

Intracavitary irradiation: As shown in Table V, the source of intracavitary irradiation in 1953 was radium only, but this has been gradually replaced by ^{60}Co and ^{137}Cs. It appears that ^{137}Cs, which is suited to the after-loading and has a longer half-life, will be used more frequently. Recently, the high dose rate intracavitary irradiation method (remote after-loading system) has been used in several hospitals, and ^{252}Cf is now also on trial.

3. Chemotherapy

Many combination therapies of anticancer drugs with surgery or radiotherapy have been carried out in many cases of carcinoma of the cervix without any fruitful conclusion.

Acknowledgment

I am greatly indebted to Dr. K. Hashimoto, Prof. Emeritus, Okayama University, Dr. S. Iwai, Chairman of the Japan Uterine Cancer Committee, and Dr. K. Masubuchi, Head of the Dept. of Gynecology, Cancer Institute Hospital, Tokyo for their guidance and encouragement over a long period.

REFERENCES

1. Hirabayashi, K., Ishikawa, K., Inoue, K., Sekiba, K., and Hashimoto, K. Prophylactic vaginal cuff irradiation in the treatment of cervical cancer by the Okabayashi operation. *Acta Obstet. Gynaecol. Japan,* **20,** 106–111 (1973).
2. Kitabatake, T. Analysis of factors influencing end results of treatment of cervical cancer in Japan, using the conception of "treatment result ratio." *Gan-no-Rinsho (Cancer Clinic),* **11,** 125–132 (1965) (in Japanese).

CANCER OF THE UTERINE CERVIX AND ENDOMETRIUM AT THE CANCER INSTITUTE HOSPITAL, TOKYO

Kazumasa Masubuchi, Shigeo Masubuchi, Hiroichi Suzumura,
Hisamitsu Kubo, Hiroyuki Okajima, Mie Ogiuchi,
Chung Duck Kim, Hsin Fu Chen, Kazuhiro Yamauchi,
and Kaoru Hattori

*Department of Gynecology, Cancer Institute Hospital**

From 1960 to 1969 a total of 2,573 patients with carcinoma of the uterine cervix and 165 patients with carcinoma of the endometrium were treated in the Cancer Institute Hospital, Tokyo, and their 5-year cure rate is reported. The correlation between the cure rate and mode of treatment is discussed.

In Stage I carcinoma of the cervix surgery gave a better result than radiation therapy. In Stage II there was no difference in cure rate between surgery and radiation therapy.

In carcinoma of the endometrium the routine treatment of choice was simple hysterectomy with bilateral salpingo-oophorectomy; this gave a fairly good result. From a recent study, the suggestion is given that pelvic lymphadenectomy should be performed routinely.

In 1949, the Department of Gynecology was established at the Cancer Institute Hospital, Tokyo. From 1950 to 1974, a total of 7,536 cases of female genital cancer were treated; carcinoma of the uterus comprised 7,102 cases (94.2%). Of 7,102 uterine carcinomata, 6,737 cases (94.9%) were carcinoma of the cervix and only 365 cases (5.1%) were carcinoma of the endometrium. The remarkably high incidence of carcinoma of the cervix and low incidence of carcinoma of the endometrium, in Japanese, are epidemiologically interesting (8).

Results obtained at this clinic have been incorporated in the "Annual Reports on the Results of Treatment in Carcinoma of the Uterus and Vagina" issued at Radium-hemmet in Stockholm (1).

In this review, the methods of treatment and the results obtained in carcinoma of the cervix and endometrium in the Cancer Institute Hospital, Tokyo, during the period of 1960–1969 are described.

Cancer of the Cervix

In the Cancer Institute Hospital during the period of 1960–1969, the method of treatment has gradually changed, especially in the field of radiotherapy. In the Stage I group, surgery gave better results rather than radiotherapy. In other stages,

* Kami-Ikebukuro 1-37-1, Toshima-ku, Tokyo 170, Japan (増淵一正, 増淵誠夫, 鈴村博一, 久保久光, 岡島弘幸, 扇内美恵, 金 貞徳, 陳 信夫, 山内一弘, 服部 香).

there was no significant difference between them. The apparatus for external irradiation has been changed from the conventional X-ray to Linac, *via* Telecobalt, during this period. Comparison of the 5-year cure rates for these three different means of radiotherapy showed that Linac gave the best result of 97% in Stage I, and the combined use of Linac and Telecobalt gave the best cure rates of 87.6% and 55.7%, respectively, for Stages II and III. Since 1967, only Linac has been used for external irradiation and several modifications in total doses and methods of application have been made.

1. Mode of treatment

During 1960–1969, a total of 2,573 patients with carcinoma of the uterine cervix were treated in the Cancer Institute Hospital, Tokyo; 1,483 of these patients were treated by radiation and the others by surgery. Five-year survival rates for each clinical stage are computed by the use of observed and expected survival rates. Since the apparatus for external irradiation has been changed during this period, the 5-year survival rates for the different types of external irradiation have also been computed.

The number of patients treated during this period is listed by stages for each year in Table I. Nearly 80% of the patients in Stage I were treated surgically. In Stage II the number of patients treated by radiotherapy was nearly the same as those by surgery. In the advanced cases, Stages III and IV, most of the patients were treated by radiotherapy. Since 1966, the patients in Stage III decreased in number, but on the other hand, those in Stages I and II gradually increased. Particularly in 1968 and 1969, the number of patients in both Stages I and II was almost twice that in Stage III. From 1968, simple hysterectomy was performed for Stage Ia cases. As will be noted from Table II, the 5-year survival rate for Stage Ia was 98.7% and no case died of the carcinoma. During this period, there was no significant increase in the 5-year

TABLE I. Number of Patients (Cervix)

Stage	Year										Total
	1960	1961	1962	1963	1964	1965	1966	1967	1968	1969	
I	88	66	64	81	82	85	65	78	96	96	801
II	118	96	89	83	66	81	104	85	95	91	908
III	107	104	92	76	91	96	67	68	51	56	808
IV	7	3	8	3	4	10	6	10	3	2	56
Total	320	269	253	243	243	272	242	241	245	245	2,573

TABLE II. Five-year Relative Survival Rate for Surgical Treatment (1960–1969) (Cervix)

	Stage I*	Stage II	Stage III	Stage IV
Number of patients	634 (70)	408	46	2
Observed survival rate (%)	92.6 (97.1)	76.4	41.3	0
Expected survival rate (%)	97.7 (98.3)	96.7	96.8	98.2
Relative survival rate (%)	94.8 (98.7)	78.3	42.7	0
Standard deviation	0.01 (0.02)	0.02	0.075	

* Figures in parentheses show number of Stage Ia (1968–1969).

TABLE III. Age Distribution for Surgical Treatment (1960–1969) (Cervix)

Age (years)	Stage I*	Stage II	Stage III	Stage IV
23–27	3	5		
28–32	34 (4)	18		
33–37	104 (12)	45	4	1
38–42	169 (22)	52	11	
43–47	118 (17)	69	7	
48–52	88 (7)	68	7	1
53–57	79 (5)	76	9	
58–62	32 (2)	60	8	
63–67	4 (1)	14		
68–72	3	1		
Total	634 (70)	408	46	2

* Figures in parenthese show number of Stage Ia (1968–1969).

TABLE IV. Five-year Relative Survival Rate for Radiotherapy (1960–1969) (Cervix)

	Stage I	Stage II	Stage III	Stage IV
Number of patients	167	500	762	54
Observed survival rate (%)	81.5	70.3	47.1	14.8
Expected survival rate (%)	93.1	91.4	92.7	93.2
Relative survival rate (%)	87.5	76.9	50.9	15.9
Standard deviation	0.032	0.022	0.019	0.052

cure rate in Stages I and II. The age distribution for the surgical group is shown in Table III.

Table IV shows the 5-year survival rate of the patients treated by radiation. Radiation treatment consisted of the combined use of intracavitary irradiation and external irradiation. During this period, only radium was applied for intracavitary irradiation. Conventional X-ray was the main apparatus for the external irradiation (Table V) at the beginning of this series, then Telecobalt took its place. In 1964, Linac was introduced and combined use of Telecobalt and Linac occurred widely during 1964–1966, giving fairly good results.

From 1967, Linac was used for all cases and resulted in a high survival rate at every stage. Table VI shows the age distribution of the patients given radiotherapy. It is obvious that the age distribution was younger in surgery than in radiotherapy.

2. Surgery versus radiotherapy

As shown in Tables II and IV, the 5-year survival rate in Stage I after surgical treatment is better than that after radiotherapy, the rates being 94.8% and 87.5%, respectively. For Stage II, the survival rate after surgery is 78.3% and that after radiotherapy is 76.9%, there being no significant difference between them. The results between surgery and radiotherapy for Stage III were almost the same. Thus, in Stage I, 634 out of 801 cases were treated surgically and fairly good results were obtained. Surgery therefore seems to be the most decisive means of cure for Stage I. In 1969, Masubuchi et al. (7) reported on 5-year cure rate with special reference to the comparison of surgical and radiation therapy, and stated that both have advantages and

TABLE V. Five-year Relative Survival Rate Classified According

| | Conventional X-ray | | | |
| | 1960–1962 | | | |
	I	II	III	I
Number of patients	32	97	112	46
Observed survival rate (%)	59.3	62.8	43.4	84.7
Expected survival rate (%)	93.5	91.3	93.4	94.5
Relative survival rate (%)	63.4	68.7	46.4	89.6
Standard deviation	0.093	0.054	0.05	0.056

TABLE VI. Age Distribution for Radiotherapy Classified According to External Radiation Apparatus (excluding Stage IV) (Cervix)

Age (years)	Conventional X-ray			Telecobalt			Combined use of Telecobalt and Linac			Linac		
	I	II	III	I	II	III	I	II	III	I	II	III
18–22			1									
23–27			1									
28–32	1		2	1		2			1			3
33–37	3	2	5	9	7	5		1	6	3	5	10
38–42	1	5	7	2	6	16	1	0	13	7	11	10
43–47	6	12	18	7	11	29	1	4	14	4	18	24
48–52	7	12	23	8	17	61	2	7	23	9	22	31
53–57	2	18	21	6	27	54	0	14	25	8	29	33
58–62	5	27	16	5	28	49	1	10	20	19	53	44
63–67	4	8	8	5	24	39	2	14	21	14	37	34
68–72	3	8	6	3	13	22	2	5	21	6	17	22
73–77		4	4		2	5	1	4	2	3	13	7
78–82		1			3				2		1	2

disadvantages. Meigs (10) reported the operability rate for Stage I as being as low as 45–60%. Curie (2) reported the results of 552 surgical operations for carcinoma of the and cervix in a 35-year period and the 5-year survival rate was 86.3% for Stage I, 75% for Stage IIa, 58.9% for Stage IIb, and 34.1% for other stages. The Stage II group can be treated virtually only by radiotherapy. We have the alternative of surgery or radiotherapy for this group but surgery cannot be applied to those whose general condition contraindicates this technique. In Stage III, only 5.6% of the cases were operated in our series with the cure rate of 42.7% and radiotherapy gave a better cure rate of 50.9%, in this group. Radiotherapy seems to be the obvious treatment of choice for Stages III and IV.

3. Five-year survival rates with different kinds of radiotherapy

During the period of 1960–1969, the apparatus for external irradiation was changed. As shown in Table V, cure rates from the conventional X-ray group were the worst for every clinical stage. It can be stated that half of the deaths in this group were not from cancer of the cervix but from some other disease (including complicato Apparatus for External Irradiation (except Stage IV) (Cervix)

Telecobalt		Combined use of Telecobalt and Linac			Linac		
1960–1966		1964–1966			1964–1969		
II	III	I	II	III	I	II	III
138	282	10	56	178	72	206	220
68.1	45.3	70.0	79.6	51.7	89.3	72.8	47.9
91.2	92.6	89.0	90.8	92.7	92.0	91.6	92.5
74.6	48.9	78.6	87.6	55.7	97.0	79.4	51.7
0.043	0.032	0.162	0.058	0.044	0.039	0.034	0.036

tions of radiotherapy, for example, rectal ulcer, bladder ulcer, fistula, or ileus, and so on). In the Telecobalt and Linac groups the main cause of death, in 85.5%, was from recurrence or metastasis of carcinoma of the uterine cervix. Comparison of the results between Telecobalt and Linac shows that the combined use of these was the best, Linac alone being second most effective. This was an unexpected result for us, because the use of Telecobalt had ended in 1967.

For intracavitary irradiation, the only source during this period was radium. The correlation between the intracavitary radium doses and the three apparatus for external irradiation is shown in Table VII.

Linac was used with the three above-mentioned means but for statistical calculation, they were collected to compare with other types of treatment in this series.

From 1970, a remote-control, after-loading system with a strong source (Ralstron) took the place of radium for intracavitary irradiation. There is no doubt that there will be much more improvement in the results of radiotherapy with the combined use of Linac and Ralstron.

TABLE VII.   Applied Doses in Radiation Treatment (Cervix)

External irradiation	Doses (rad) to point B	Intracavitary radium (mgh)	
		ovoid	tandem
Conventional X-ray	1,200 or 1,500	3,450	2,760
Telecobalt	4,000 or 5,000	3,450	27,60
Combined use of Telecobalt and Linac	2,000 (Telecobalt) 3,000[a] (Linac)	2,300	1,840
Linac	3,000 or 5,000	3,600	2,400
Linac	3,000[a] plus 2,000	2,300	1,840

[a] Whole pelvis irradiation; others, with central shielding.

4. Conclusion

From 1960 to 1969, a total of 2,573 patients with cancer of the uterine cervix were treated in the Cancer Institute Hospital, Tokyo. In Stage I, surgery seems to be better than radiotherapy. In Stage II, surgery and radiotherapy gave nearly the same 5-year cure rates. In other stages, radiotherapy was the obvious treatment of choice. Recently, the instruments for radiotherapy, both intracavitary and external irradiation, have been improved and there is no doubt that the 5-year cure rates will continue to improve.

Cancer of the Endometrium

The rate of corpus cancer in uterine cancer as a whole is reported to be 20–30% in Europe and the United States, but the rate is low in Japan, being only 2–5%. In recent years, the incidence of corpus cancer has increased to about 10% of the whole of uterine cancer as in the Department of Gynecology, Cancer Institute Hospital, Tokyo, reported by Masubuchi and others (*9*).

This study includes 165 patients with a diagnosis of invasive endometrial adeno-carcinoma during 1960–1969. Patients with adenomatous hyperplasia or carcinoma *in situ* of the endometrium, are excluded. Full follow-up information was obtained in 164 cases for 5 years and only one case was lost to follow-up before this period.

1. Evaluation of survival rate

To examine the results of the treatment, the 5-year survival rate was used and this was calculated using the life table method (*3*). According to the classification of the International Federation of Obstetrics and Gynecology (FIGO), these 165 cases were classified into 132 cases of Stage I, 11 of Stage II, 16 of Stage III, and 6 of Stage IV. The incidence of Stage I is very high (80%) and a similar finding was reported by other investigators (*4–6, 15*). During the 5 years after treatment, 30 patients died and one case was lost to follow-up. Therefore, the total observed 5-year survival rate based on all stages of endometrial carcinoma was 81.8% and the relative survival rate was 88.3%. It is usually considered that the prognosis for corpus carcinoma is good, and many reports showed a high rate of 5-year survival (*4–6, 12, 13, 15*). Table VIII shows the stage distribution of patients and their 5-year survival rate.

Among these 30 dead patients, 19 were in Stage I, 1 in Stage II, 4 in Stage III, and 6 in Stage IV, and 24 had died within 2 years after the treatment. A similar result

TABLE VIII. Five-year Survival Rate of Each Clinical Stage (Endometrium)

Stage	No. of patients	No. of dead within 5-years	Lost to follow-up	Observed 5-year survival (%)	Relative 5-year survival (%)	Standard deviation
I	132	19		85.6	92.2	0.033
II	11	1		90.9	96.6	0.092
III	16	4	1	73.9	80.6	0.120
IV	6	6		0	0	
Total	165	30				

TABLE IX. Age Distribution and Survival (Endometrium)

Age (years)	No. of patients	No. of deaths	5-Year survival (%)
–39	5	1	80
40–49	30	2	93.3
50–59	67	8	88.1
60–69	50	14	72.0
70–	13	5	61.5
Total	165	30	

TABLE X. Subclassification of Stage I and Survival Rate (Endometrium)

Stage	No. of patients	No. of deaths	Observed 5-year survival (%)
Ia	81	12	85.2
Ib	51	7	86.3

was reported by Homesley and others (5). The age distribution of these patients is shown in Table IX.

In 1970, the new FIGO classification divided the earlier Stage I into subgroups according to the size of the uterus. According to this new FIGO classification, 132 cases of Stage I were divided into subgroups Ia and Ib retrospectively based on the operative and clinical findings. The difference in 5-year survival rate between Stages Ia and Ib was not statistically significant (Table X).

A total of 165 patients ranged in age from 26 to 82 years, 160 patients being more than 40 years of age (97%), with a peak occurrence of the disease in the 60s and 70s. The mean age was 56.4 years.

A study of the relation of age to survival indicates that survival is inversely proportional to increasing age; similar findings have been reported by others (11, 14, 15).

2. Mode of treatment

For the treatment of endometrial carcinoma, the majority of 161 patients were treated by surgery, with or without other combined therapy, and only 4 cases were treated by radiation, because of the intercurrent disease or a technically inoperable condition.

The main treatment method used in this period for endometrial carcinoma was total abdominal simple hysterectomy with a vaginal cuff and bilateral salpingo-oophorectomy; 113 patients were treated by this method. The 5-year survival rate after this method was 86.7%. Seventeen patients were treated by hysterectomy and postoperative external irradiation and 22 patients were treated by operation and progesterone therapy. Nine patients were treated by radical hysterectomy with pelvic lymphadenectomy and

TABLE XI. Method of Therapy and Survival (Endometrium)

Stage	Method of therapy	No. of patients	No. of deaths 0-1	1-2	2-3	3-4	4-5	Total No.	5-Year survival (%)
			(years after treatment)						
I	Hysterectomy	98	2	5	2	1	1	11	88.8
	+radiation	9	3	1	0	0	0	4	55.5
	+progesterone	20	1	1	0	0	0	3	85.0
	Radical hysterectomy	4	0	0	0	0	0	0	100
	Radiation	1	1	0	0	0	0	1	0
II–IV	Hysterectomy	15	3	1	0	0	0	4	73.3
	+radiation	8	1	2	0	1	0	4	50.0
	+progesterone	2	1	0	0	0	0	1	50.0
	Radical hysterectomy	5	0	0	0	0	0	0	100
	Radiation (1 lost to follow-up)	3	1	1	0	0	0	2	0

TABLE XII. Myometrial Invasion and Survival in Stage I (Endometrium)

Grade of invasion	No. of patients	5-Year survival	
		No.	%
Confined to endometrium only	18	16	88.8
Myometrial invasion			
Slight	75	63	84.0
Moderate	20	17	85.0
Deep	18	13	72.2

these 9 patients were all healthy 5 years after the treatment. The result of these treatments is shown in Table XI.

Sall and others (*14*) showed that involvement of the cervix in endometrial carcinoma resulted in a poor prognosis (50% 5-year survival rate) but, in the present study, prognosis of Stage II endometrial carcinoma was fairly good.

Stage I endometrial carcinoma is defined as a carcinoma confined to the corpus. This means that there may be cases with or without myometrial invasion. Stage I lesions are subdivided according to the depth of myometrial invasion. The correlation between the myometrial invasion and 5-year survival in Stage I is shown in Table XII. In 93 cases out of 131 operated cases of Stage I, carcinoma involved the endometrium only or a slight depth of myometrium, and in 38 cases carcinoma involved a moderate depth or more of the myometrium, but between these 2 groups the difference in 5-year survival rate was not significant.

The most important factor which relates to the cure rate is the histological finding. Cases with poorly differentiated adenocarcinoma especially with the anaplastic type of carcinoma gave a poor cure rate. Fortunately, the anaplastic type of carcinoma occurs infrequently. In this study, out of 165 cases only 15 cases were of the anaplastic type.

3. Present and future aspects of carcinoma of the endometrium in Japan

As already stated, the incidence of endometrial carcinoma in Japan used to be low but, according to changes in dietary habits and in living conditions, this incidence has been showing a relatively rapid increase in the last 10 years. This tendency will continue in the future in Japan.

At present, the routine treatment of choice in this clinic for carcinoma of the endometrium is simple hysterectomy with bilateral salpingo-oophorectomy and with pelvic lymphadenectomy. In the past, it was thought that pelvic lymph node metastasis was quite rare in endometrial carcinoma, but recent data in this clinic show that positive nodes are not so rare. Therefore, the importance of pelvic node dissection in endometrial carcinoma should be emphasized.

REFERENCES

1. Annual Report on the Results of Treatment in Carcinoma of the Uterus. Radiumhemmet, Stockholm, Vol. 12–15 (1961–1976).
2. Curie, D. W. Operative treatment of cancer of the cervix. *J. Obstet. Gynaecol. Br. Commun.*, **78**, 385–405 (1971).
3. Cutler, S. J. Computation of survival. *Natl. Cancer Inst. Monogr.*, **15**, 381–385 (1964).

4. Gusberg, S. B. and Yannopoulos, D. Therapeutic decisions in corpus cancer. *Am. J. Obstet. Gynecol.*, **88**, 157–162 (1964).

5. Hemesley, H., Boronow, R., and Lewis, J., Jr. Treatment of adenocarcinoma of the endometrium at Memorial-James Ewing Hospitals, 1949–1965. *Obstet. Gynecol.*, **47**, 100–105 (1976).

6. Karlstedt, K. Carcinoma of the uterine corpus: Factors bearing on the curability. *Acta Radiol. (Suppl.)*, **282**, 1–98 (1968).

7. Masubuchi, K., Tenjin, Y., Kubo, H., and Kimura, M. Five-year cure rate for carcinoma of the cervix uteri, with special reference to the comparison of surgical and radiation therapy. *Am. J. Obstet. Gynecol.*, **103**, 566–573 (1969).

8. Masubuchi, K. and Nemoto, H. Epidemiologic studies on uterine cancer at the Cancer Institute Hospital, Tokyo, Japan. *Cancer*, **30**, 268–275 (1972).

9. Masubuchi, K., Nemoto, H., Masubuchi, S., Fujimoto, I., and Uchino, S. Increasing incidence of endometrial carcinoma in Japan. *Gynecol. Oncol.*, **3**, 335–346 (1975).

10. Meigs, J. V. "Surgical Treatment of Cancer of Cervix," Grune & Stratton, New York, pp. 192–196 (1954).

11. Milton, P.J.D. and Metters, J. S. Endometrial carcinoma: An analysis of 355 cases treated at St. Thomas' Hospital, 1945–69. *J. Obstet. Gynaecol. Br. Commun.*, **79**, 455–464 (1972).

12. Ng, A.B.D. and Reagan, J. W. Incidence and prognosis of endometrial carcinoma by histologic grade and extent. *Obstet. Gynecol.*, **35**, 437–443 (1970).

13. Nieminen, U. and Soderlin, E. Results of the treatment of carcinoma of the corporis uteri. *Strahlentherapie*, **143**, 159–163 (1972).

14. Sall, S., Sonnenblick, B., and Stone, M. Factors affecting survival of patients with endometrial adenocarcinoma. *Am. J. Obstet. Gynecol.*, **107**, 116–123 (1970).

15. Soderlin, E. Factors affecting prognosis of endometrial carcinoma. *Acta Obstet. Gynecol. Scand. (Suppl.)*, **38**, 5–37 (1974).

GANN Monograph on Cancer Research 22, 1979

CANCER OF THE OVARY

Shoichi HACHIYA and Yoshiteru TERASHIMA

*Department of Obstetrics and Gynecology, Jikei
University School of Medicine**

The treatment of ovarian cancer has scarcely improved over the past 30 years. The reasons for poor prognosis are these: 1) The early diagnosis is difficult, 2) various kinds of tumors can be seen in the ovary, and 3) there are no established therapies for these tumors. The results of treatment of ovarian cancers should be compared for the same stage-grouping and histological classification. From this point the International Federation of Gynecology and Obstetrics (FIGO) stage-grouping and histological classification are acknowledged significant in this study.

Prognosis is poor in primary ovarian carcinoma, the 5-year survival rate being only 21.8%, and that in Stage Ia 58.3%; thus, intensive postoperative therapy is desirable. The 5-year survival rate in Stage Ic is also only 36.8%, suggesting the previous dissemination of the cancer cells in the peritoneal cavity; therefore, these cases should be treated in the same way as Stages II and III.

Prognosis is relatively favorable in low potential malignancy, the 5-year survival rate being 85.7%, and the 10-year survival rate, 71.4%. Furthermore, even the 5-year survival rate in Stage II cases is 77.3%.

The anaplastic serous and undifferentiated carcinomata often have a poor prognosis.

The 5-year survival rate in dysgerminoma, being 72.3%, is relatively high, while prognosis is very poor in embryonal carcinoma having the same origin of germ cell, about 95% of cases terminating fatally within 1 year, and the 2-year survival rate being only 13.1%.

Despite the marked progress in the diagnosis and treatment of uterine cancer and chorionic tumors, little improvement has been achieved in the results of treatment for ovarian malignancies during the past 30 years. The following may be the reasons:

1) That the early diagnosis of these malignancies is difficult.
2) That many kinds of tumors are included in ovarian malignancies, and vary in prognosis.
3) That there are no established therapies for these malignancies.

Difficulty in early diagnosis: Named "silent disease" or "creeping disease," about 80% of cancers of the ovary had already extended into the pelvic and peritoneal cavity at laparotomy, and this has not altered for the past 30 years (Table I).

Classification of malignant ovarian tumors: "Cancer of the ovary" commonly includes not only adenocarcinoma of surface epithelial origin, but also malignant tumors derived

* Nishi-Shinbashi 3-25-8, Minato-ku, Tokyo 105, Japan (蜂屋祥一, 寺島芳輝).

TABLE I. Stage of Ovarian Cancer Laparotomy

Author	Year	Within the ovary		Beyond the ovary	
		Number of cases	%	Number of cases	%
Montgomery	1948	18	26.5	50	73.5
Taylor	1959	56	29.0	137	71.0
Turner	1959	39	22.7	128	77.3
Rubin	1962	23	15.8	122	84.2
Dockerty	1962	38	23.1	126	76.9
Higuchi	1970	35	20.6	135	79.4

TABLE II. Ovarian Malignancy and Prognosis

Kind of tumor	Prognosis
1. Surface epithelial tumors	5-Year survival, 85%
1) Malignancy with low potential	10-Year survival, 70%
Serous, mucinous, endometrioid, mesonephric cystadenomas with proliferating activity of the epithelial cells and nuclear abnormalities but with no infiltrative destructive growth	5-Year survival of patients in Stages II and III, 70%
2) Serous cystadenocarcinomas Mucinous cystadenocarcinomas Endometrioid adenocarcinomas Mesonephroid cystadenocarcinomas Concominant carcinomas ; undifferentiated carcinoma. Tumors composed of a mixture of two or more of the four types described above ; a malignant tumor of epithelial structure that is too poorly differentiated to be placed in any of the four groups above.	Relatively more favorable in mucinous, endometrioid, and mesonephroid type than in serous and undifferentiated type
2. Germ cell origin tumors	
1) Dysgerminoma	5-Year survival, about 80% Relatively good (poor in some cases)
2) Extraembryonal tumors Chorioepithelioma Endodermal sinus tumor (yolk sac tumor)	Extremely poor (2-year survival less than 10%)
3) Embryonal tumors (carcinoma)	
Teratoma {immature intermediate mature	Poor Relatively good Good
4) Mixed embryonal and extraembryonal tumors	Extremely poor
3. Sex cord mesenchyme tumors	
1) Granulosa-theca cell tumor	
2) Sertoli-Leydig cell tumor {well differentiated intermediate undifferentiated	5-Year survival of about 80%, relatively good
(Arrhenoblastoma Androblastoma)	
4. Stromal tumors sartoma	Poor
5. Metastic tumors	Poor

from the germ cell, the sex cord mesenchyme, and stroma, which differ in prognosis from each other (Table II).

Current status of treatment of cancer of the ovary: Many studies on the treatment of ovarian cancer are reported, but a review of these papers indicates the following:

   a) The results of treatment often vary in studies, and have not been improved.
   b) They do not always demonstrate treatment of the same types of tumors.
   c) There are many different methods of treatment for ovarian cancer.

Treatment of Carcinoma of the Ovary

It is of the utmost importance for the method of treatment to determine the extent of the tumor (stage-grouping) in laparotomy and histological features.

1. Stage-grouping

The results of treatment should be reported according to the stage-grouping in laparotomy which was proposed by the International Federation of Gynecology and Obstetrics (FIGO) (Table III).

TABLE III. Stage-grouping for Primary Carcinoma of the Ovary

Stage I	Growth limited to the ovaries
Stage Ia	Growth limited to one ovary; no ascites,
	(i) No tumor on the external surface; capsule intact
	(ii) Tumor present on the external surface or/and capsule ruptured
Stage Ib	Growth limited to both ovaries; no ascites
	(i) No tumor on the external surface; capsule intact
	(ii) Tumor present on the external surface or/and capsule ruptured
Stage Ic	Tumor either Stage Ia or Stage Ib, but with ascites present or positive peritoneal washings
Stage II	Growth involving one or both ovaries with pelvic extension
Stage IIa	Extension and/or metastases to the uterus and/or tubes
Stage IIb	Extension to other pelvic tissues including the peritoneum
Stage IIc	Tumor either Stage IIa or Stage IIb, but with ascites present or positive peritoneal washings
Stage III	Growth involving one or both ovaries with intraperitoneal metastases outside the pelvis and/or positive retroperitoneal nodes. Tumor limited to the true pelvis with histologically proven malignant extention to small bowel or omentum
Stage IV	Growth involving one or both ovaries with distant metastases. If there is pleural effusion there must be positive cytology to allot a case to Stage IV. Parenchymal liver metastases equal Stage IV.

Based on findings at clinical examination and surgical exploration. The final histology after surgery is to be considered in the staging, as is cytology as far as effusion is concerned. Ascites is peritoneal effusion which in the opinion of the surgeon is pathological or/and clearly exceeds nomal amounts.

2. Type of tumor

Granulosa cell tumor and dysgerminoma, have often been reported as "cancer of the ovary," which may be one of the reasons why the results of treatment have varied vastly between institutions. In the future, the treatment of ovarian cancer should be discussed in terms of the same stage and histological pattern.

Germ cell origin tumors such as dysgerminoma, teratoma, embryonal carcinoma, and chorioepithelioma vary widely in prognosis, hence, it is necessary to examine the tumors histologically in detail.

Granulosa cell tumor and Sertoli-Leydig cell tumor (Arrhenoblastoma) produce estrogen or androgen to present their characteristic manifestations, but their prognosis is relatively favorable, the 5-year survival rate being about 80% (Table II).

3. Histological classification of the common primary epithelial tumors of the ovary

FIGO classified the tumors derived from the surface epithelium into 5 groups, and further divided each of the groups into 3 subgroups, *i.e.*, benign cystomas, low potential malignancy, and cystadenocarcinoma. It is true that there yet remain problems to be solved in the criteria of mesonephroid tumor and low potential malignancy; however, it is important to report the treatment of the common primary epithelial tumors of the ovary according to this classification (Table IV).

TABLE IV. Histological Classification of the Common Primary Epithelial Tumors of the Ovary

I. Serous cystomas
   a) Serous benign cystadenomas
   b) Serous cystadenomas with proliferating activity of the epithelial cells and nuclear abnormalities but with no infiltrative destructive growth (borderline cases ; low potential malignancy)
   c) Serous cystadenocarcinomas
II. Mucinous cystomas
   a) Mucinous benign cystadenomas
   b) Mucinous cystadenomas with proliferating activity of the epithelial cells and nuclear abnormalities but with no infiltrative destructive growth (borderline cases ; low potential malignancy)
   c) Mucinous cystadenocarcinomas
III. Endometrioid tumors (similar to adenocarcinomas in the endometrium)
   a) Benign endometriod cysts
   b) Endometrioid tumors with proliferating activity of the epithelial cells and nuclear abnormalities but with no infiltrative destructive growth (borderline cases ; low potential malignancy)
   c) Endometrioid adenocarcinomas
IV. Mesonephroid tumors (clear cell tumors)
   a) Benign mesonephroid tumors
   b) Mesonephroid tumors with proliferating activity of the epithelial cells and nuclear abnormalities but with no infiltrative destructive growth (borderline cases ; low potential malignancy)
   c) Mesonephroid cystadenocarcinomas
V. Concomitant carcinomas, unclassified carcinoma (tumors which cannot be allotted to one of the groups I, II, III, or IV)
      Concominant carcinoma ; undifferentiated carcinoma. Tumors composed of a mixture of two or more of the four types described above ; a malignant tumor of epithelial structure that is too poorly differentiated to be placed in any of the four groups above.
VI. No histology

Treatment of Ovarian Cancer in Our Department

All cases of ovarian cancer are first histologically examined, and then treated in our department.

1.   Treatment of early cancer (Stage I)
Surgical therapy: Total hysterectomy and bilateral salpingo-oophorectomy are performed, and omentectomy is also performed in cases of embryonal carcinoma and undifferentiated carcinoma. Low potential malignancy, dysgerminoma, immature teratoma, and granulosa cell tumor are indications for conservative operation. This operation should be performed only in Stage Ia, but cases of radical operation should be performed.

Conservative operation should also be clinically confined to puberty and young women who have no children, while the radical operation should be performed in menopause or in women who do not desire to have a child. However, it has been reported that invasion and metastasis are found in about 10% of early cancers. For this reason, a scraping smear should be performed on the tumor capsule, cul-de-sac, omentum, and mesentery; the other ovary should be carefully examined even if normal in size, and if any abnormality is found consequently, wedge resection should be performed.
Adjuvant therapy: In almost all cases, radical operation for early cancer is followed by radiotherapy or chemotherapy.

Postoperative therapy is performed, partly for prophylactic purposes, against microinvasions and metastases which cannot be detected, and no improvement in treatment of ovarian cancer can be expected without combination therapy. Intraperitoneal administration of anticancer agents or ^{198}Au colloid, irradiation with the linear accelerator, and chemotherapy are employed as adjuvant therapy.

2.   Treatment of advanced cancer
Surgical therapy: If the tumor has spread widely in the pelvic and peritoneal cavity (Stages II, III, and VI), the operation should be confined only to exploratory laparotomy; intensive chemotherapy should be immediately performed to improve the general condition and regress the tumor; at the second look operation, the tumor should be resected wherever possible.

In cases presenting a marked invasion into the Douglas' cul-de-sac, the uterus may be left unresected to use it as the applicator for radium.
Radiation therapy: The whole abdominal irradiation used to be performed as radiation therapy, however digestive disturbances such as ileus, abdominal pain due to adhesion, diarrhea, and blooded stools were often complaints. Therefore, Stage III cancer recently has been treated by chemotherapy, and Stage II cancers chiefly are irradiated by anterior and posterior 2-field irradiation with the 6 V linear accelerator, CD of 1 m, 200 rad per fraction, 5 times a week, up to total dose of 5,000 rad and over the 15×16 cm area of pelvic cavity from the L_4 as the upper margin to the pubic symphysis.
Chemotherapy: There are many anticancer agents, but multiple combination chemotherapy by means of intraperitoneal, intravenous, and continuous intra-arterial infusion have chiefly been employed.

FAMT therapy with 500 mg 5-fluorouracil (5-FU), 200 mg of cyclophosphamide, 2 mg of mitmycin C (MMC), and 0.5 mg of Toyomycin simultaneously, twice or 3 times a week by the intravenous route, not less than 12 times, has chiefly been employed. However, recently, combination therapy with 3 mg of carboquone (CQ), 500 mg of 5-FU, and 40 mg of cytosine arabinoside simultaneously, twice a week (CQ by

TABLE V-A. Stage and 5-Year Survival Rate in Primary Ovarian Carcinoma

	Stage	Number of cases	%	5-Year survival	
				Number of survivals	%
Early cancer	Ia	12 ⎫		7	58.3
	b	4 ⎬ 35	20.6	2	50.0
	c	19 ⎭		7	36.8
Advanced cancer	IIa	6 ⎫		2	33.3
	b	40 ⎬ 135	79.4	9	22.5
	III	87		10	11.5
	IV	2 ⎭		0	0
Total		170		37	21.8

TABLE V-B.

Years of observation	Alive at beginning of interval	Died during interval	Lost to follow-up during interval	With-drawn alive during interval	Effective number exposed to the risk of dying	Propor-tion dying	Propor-tion surviving	Cumulative proportion surviving
$X-L \sim X$	LX	DX	UX	WX	$\dfrac{L'X}{LX-1/2(UX+WX)}$	$\dfrac{QX}{DX/L'X}$	$\dfrac{PX}{L-QX}$	$\dfrac{PX}{P_1P_2...PX}$
0–1	345	102	32	3	327.5	0.311	0.689	0.689
1–2	208	49	—	5	205.5	0.238	0.762	0.525
2–3	154	25	—	7	141.5	0.177	0.823	0.432
3–4	122	14	—	7	118.5	0.118	0.882	0.381
4–5	101	7	—	11	95.5	0.073	0.927	0.353
5–	74	9	—	65				

LX, alive at beginning of interval; DX, died during interval; UX, lost to follow-up during interval; WX, withdrawn alive during interval; L'X, effective number exposed to the risk of dying; QX, proportion dying; PX, proportion surviving.

TABLE V-C.

	1-Year rate	5-Year rate
Observed survival rate	0.689	0.353
Expected survival rate	0.936	0.892
Relative survival rate	0.736	0.395
	73.6%	39.5%
Standard deviation		
1-Year rate	$\sigma r = \sqrt{\dfrac{0.689(1-0.689)}{345}}\Big/0.936 = 0.027$	
5-Year rate	$\sigma r = \sqrt{\dfrac{0.353(1-0.353)}{345}}\Big/0.892 = 0.029$	

intravenous one-shot injection), over 4 to 5 weeks, has chiefly been performed.

Methotrexate (MTX) and actinomycin D may be used in embryonal carcinoma and chorioepithelioma.

TABLE VI. Five-year Survival in Malignancy with Low Potential

Stage	Number of cases		5-Year survival rate	
			Number of survivals	%
I a	14⎫		14⎫	
b	0⎬ 20		0⎬ 19	95.0
c	6⎭		5⎭	
II a	2⎫		2⎫	
b	5⎪ 22		4⎪ 17	77.3
III	15⎪		11⎪	
IV	0⎭		0⎭	
Total	42		36	85.7

Death after 5 years in 6 cases, 10-year survival rate; 71.4%.

Results of Treatment of Cancer of the Ovary

1. Common primary epithelial tumors of the ovary

Stage and prognosis: Two hundred and twelve cases were histologically divided into 42 cases of low potential malignancy and 170 of primary ovarian carcinoma (Tables V-A, V-B, V-C, and VI). As expected, prognosis becomes poorer as the stage advances. Only one-half of patients in Stage Ia and Ib, and 7 of 19 patients in Stage Ic (36.8%) survived for 5 years. These figures are similar to those for patients in Stage II.

As one of the reasons for such poor prognosis, the rate of confinement of cancer within the ovary can be implicated; thus the confinement is found in 35 cases of early cancer (Stage I), representing only 20%, while extraovarian spread accounts for about 80%; and intraperitoneal metastasis (Stage III) is twice as frequent as intrapelvic metastasis (Stage II). It is, however, noteworthy, that even in advanced cancer at Stage II and III, long-term survival occured in 21 of 135 cases (15.6%). Histological features and the method of treatment thus appear to influence the prognosis.

Five-year survival of 36 of 42 cases of low potential malignancy (85.7%) indicates

TABLE VII. Five-year Survival in Each Histological Type

Histological type		Number of cases	5-Year survival	
			Number of survivals	%
Serous	b	20	17	85.0
	c	42	5	11.9
Mucinous	b	22	19	86.4
	c	71	22	31.0
Endometrioid	b	0	0	
	c	7	4	57.1
Mesonephroid	b	0	0	
	c	10	2	20.0
Undifferentiated		40	4	10.0
Total		212	73	34.4

a much better prognosis than ovarian cancer. Six more died after 5 years, giving a 10-year survival of 71.4% (Table VI).

Histologic classification and prognosis: Five-year survival in patients with each histological type of adenocarcinoma was 22 of 71 (31.0%) of the mucinous type, and 4 of 7 (57.1%) of the endometrioid type, suggesting a relatively favorable prognosis.

Prognosis in the serous and undifferentiated types, on the other hand, was extremely poor, with a 5-year survival rate of 11.9 and 10.0%, respectively, in agreement with past reports.

TABLE VIII-A. Stage of Dysgerminoma Ovarii and 5-Year Survival Rate

Stage	Number of cases	Frequency (%)	5-Year survival	
			Number of cases	Survival rate (%)
I a	32	34.0	28	81.3
b	—	—	—	—
c	30	31.9	25	83.3
II a	1	1.1	1	
b	16	17.1	9	56.3
III	15	15.9	7	46.7
IV	—	—	—	—
Total	94	100.0	68	72.3

TABLE VIII-B.

Year of observation	Alive at beginning of interval	Died during interval	Lost to follow-up during interval	Withdrawn alive during interval	Effective number exposed to the risk of dying	Proportion dying	Proportion surviving (1—Col. 7)	Cumulative proportion surviving
$X-L\sim X$	LX	DX	LLX	WX	L' LX$-1/2$ (UX+WX)	QX DX/L'X	PX L$-$QX	PX $P_1P_2...PX$
0–	153	13	29	1	138	0.094	0.906	0.906
1–	110	4	—	3	108.5	0.037	0.963	0.872
2–	103	4	—	3	101.5	0.039	0.961	0.838
3–	96	10	—	5	93.5	0.107	0.893	0.749
4–	81	2	—	3	79.5	0.025	0.975	0.730
5–	76	6	—	70				

TABLE VIII-C.

	1-Year rate	5-Year rate
Observed survival rate	0.906	0.730
Expected survival rate	0.998	0.988
Relative survival rate	0.908	0.739

Standard deviation

1-Year rate $\qquad \sigma r = \sqrt{\dfrac{0.906\,(1-0.906)}{153}}\Big/ 0.998 = 0.024$

5-Year rate $\qquad \sigma r = \sqrt{\dfrac{0.730\,(1-0.730)}{153}}\Big/ 0.988 = 0.036$

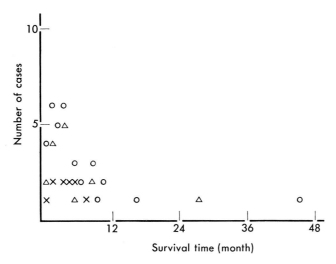

FIG. 1. Distribution of survival period in 63 fatal cases of ovarian embryonal carcinoma

○ A group; △ B group (A+dysgerminoma); × C group (A+teratoma).

Prognosis was favorable in low potential malignancy as described above, and 6 cases of fatal outcome after 5 years might indicate a relatively slow course of this tumor, pointing out the need for long-term follow-up (Table VII).

2. Germ cell origin tumors

Dysgerminoma: There were 62 Stage I (66.0%) out of 94 dysgerminoma, while Stage I accounted for only 31.1% of embryonal carcinomas. The 5-year survival rate was 80% at Stage I. As the stage advanced, the prognosis tended to be poorer. However, attention should be called to the finding that a 5-year survival rate was achieved in about 50% of Stage III (Tables VIII-A, VIII-B, and VIII-C).

Embryonal carcinoma: Sixty (95%) of the 63 cases of embryonal carcinoma terminated fatally within 1 year, 3 after 1 year but within 5 years, and none after 5 years of survival (Fig. 1). We employ a 2-year survival rate for prognosis of embryonal carcinoma. Group A consists of embryonal carcinoma, and group B and C consist of the mixed

TABLE IX-A. Stage of Ovarian Embryonal Carcinoma and 2-Year Survival Rate

Stage	Number of cases	Frequency (%)	2-Year survivals	
			Number of survivals	%
Ia	7⎫		4⎫	
b	1⎬ 19	31.1	0⎬ 8	42.1
c	11⎭		4⎭	
IIa	0⎫		0	
b	14⎬ 14	22.9	0	
III	27	44.2	0	
IV	1	1.8	0	
Total	61	100	8	13.1

TABLE IX-B.

Year of observation	Alive at beginning of interval	Died during interval	Lost to follow-up during interval	With-drawn alive during interval	Effective number exposed to the risk of dying	Proportion dying	Proportion surviving	Cumulative proportion surviving
$X-L\sim X$	LX	DX	LLX	WX	L' $LX-1/2$ $(UX+WX)$	QX $DX/L'X$	PX $L-QX$	PX $P_1P_2...PX$
0–	117	75	21	—	106.5	0.704	0.296	0.296
1–	21	3	4	—	19	0.157	0.842	0.249
2–	14	3	1	—	13.5	0.222	0.778	0.194
3–	10	1	—	—	10	0.1	0.9	0.175
4–	9	—	—	—	9	0	1	0.175
5–	9			9				

TABLE IX-C.

	1-Year rate	5-Year rate
Observed survival rate	0.296	0.175
Expected survival rate	0.998	0.992
Relative survival rate	0.297	0.176
Standard deviation		
1-Year rate	$\sigma r = \sqrt{0.001781}/0.998 = 0.423$	
5-Year rate	$\sigma r = \sqrt{0.0012339}/0.992 = 0.035$	

types. Group B is embryonal and dysgerminoma, and Group C is the cases of embryonal carcinoma and teratoma.

Prognosis is extremely poor, a 2-year survival rate having been achieved in only eight (13.1%) of 61 cases. The survivals belonged to Stage I. Stage II and III accounted for about 70% of the 61 cases, but there were no 2-year survivals (Tables IX-A, IX-B, and IX-C).

Immature teratoma varies vastly in prognosis. It is common that prognosis greatly depends on the histologic features, and often prognosis is poor in cases presenting an immature tissue which includes the nerve tissue.

REFERENCES

1. Montgomery, J. B. Malignant tumor of the ovary. *Am. J. Obstet. Gynecol.*, **55**, 201–217 (1948).
2. Rubin, P. A critical analysis of current therapy of carcinoma of the ovary. *Am. J. Roentgenol.*, **88**, 833–840 (1962).
3. Taylor, H. C. Studies on the clinical and biological evaluation of adenocarcinoma of the ovary. *J. Obstet. Gynaecol. Br. Commun.*, **66**, 827–842 (1959).
4. Turner, J. C., ReMine, W. H., and Dockerty, M. B. A clinicopathologic study of 172 patients with primary carcinoma of the ovary. *Surg. Gynecol. Obstet.*, **109**, 198–206 (1959).

CANCER OF THE BREAST IN JAPAN

Masao FUJIMORI

*Saitama Cancer Center**

We have witnessed a gradual increase, in Japan, in deaths due to breast cancer since the beginning of the 1960's. Up to the 1960's a marked improvement had been seen in the results of our treatment of breast cancer. However, at that time we appeared to enter a stalemate phase with no notable improvement since then. Early cancer (Stage I, TNM of UICC) recurrence rates stand at about 9% with a majority of the cases due to hematogenic metastasis. As to treatment methods, surgery accounts for the vast majority of cases, with a decline in the use of radiotherapy and an increase in chemotherapy constituting the current trend.

However, we are still without what might be called an epoch-making, effective anticancer agent. Further, it would appear that we cannot be too confident of continued improvement in survival rate through employment of postoperative radiotherapy.

The 5- and 10-year relative survival rate (R.S.R.) seen in 2,145 cases treated during the 1960's by our research group on "The Choice of Treatment for Breast Cancer (RGCTBC)" supported by the Ministry of Health and Welfare, stands, respectively, at 79.2% and 68.6%. In either instance, this was a higher rate than that seen in Norway and in the U.S.A. In the 5-year R.S.R. sector no significant difference was observed between cases treated by typical radical mastectomy and those treated by modified radical mastectomy.

We still remain at a loss as to the vital details dictating the selection and combination of methods of treatment during each clinical stage of breast cancer: Surgery (radical mastectomy, modified radical mastectomy, simple mastectomy), radiotherapy, chemotherapy, and hormonal therapy. Although breast cancer, in Japan, was not a major problem in the past, the current gradual increase heightens our need to find a solution. Based on my 30 years of study of breast cancer, and on my role in the organization of the above-mentioned RGCTBC in 1955, as well as the establishment of the Japan Mammary Cancer Society and the Japan Committee on TNM Classification of Breast Cancer of UICC, both in 1964, I should like to introduce the results of breast cancer treatment in Japan during the 1960's.

Review of Results of Breast Cancer Treatment before 1960

Results of breast cancer treatment were shown in terms of crude survival rate before 1960. At the same time, the clinical stages of breast cancer appeared under

---

* Komuro 818, Ina-machi, Saitama 362, Japan (藤森正雄).

Steinthal's or Portmann's classification, not according to TNM classification of UICC. Again, during this period there was no nationwide, united report of the results of breast cancer treatment in Japan. Reporting was done separately by the various hospitals involved. For our purposes ,we will review the results of treatment at the following representative institutions: Tokyo University Hospital, Cancer Institute Hospital, and the Mitsui Charity Hospital (present-day Mitsui Memorial Hospital).

Five-year crude survival rates stood at 37.9% for 36/95 cases (1923–1932 as reported by Saeiki (10)) at Tokyo University Hospital; 60.8% for 59/97 cases (1946–1951, Kajitani (10)) at the Cancer Institute Hospital and 72.2% for 57/79 cases (1948–1960, Fujimori (5)) at the Mitsui Charity Hospital. However, attention is directed here to the respective clinical Stage I (Steinthal) 81.8%, 80.0%, and 80.9% 5-year survival rates which compare well with results obtained nowadays.

Viewed in terms of the distribution of the clinical stages at which patients received treatment, we find Stage I treatment at the three institutions reported, respectively, as 11.6%, 58.5% and 26.6%. Stage III patients appear at 15.8%, 3.5%, and 21.5%. Here, we would further note that the percentage of early stage treatment of patients was lower than that pertaining today.

Increase in Numbers of Breast Cancer Deaths in Japan

In the past deaths due to breast cancer were not numerous. Unfortunately, however, the trend today is a gradual increase in breast cancer mortalities. For example, the number of breast cancer deaths (female) stood at 1,446 in 1952, 1,740 in 1962, and 2,762 in 1972. That is, an increase at the rate of 1.2 times during the 10-year period from 1952 to 1962; this rose to 1.59 during the decade 1962–1972.

Studying the period of 1952–1962 in terms of the ratio of increase in cancer death causes in Japanese women, we find lung cancer in first place with a 3.85-fold increase over the previous decade, followed by pancreatic cancer (3.41), leukemia (2.05), and breast cancer ranked sixth with a 1.2-fold increase over the previous 10 years. In the subsequent 10 years (1962–1972), however, breast cancer deaths rose to second place with an increase ratio of 1.59 over that for the previous decade. The first place is occupied by pancreatis cancer (2.12), with the lung cnacer death rate ratio falling to third place (1.47) (Hirayama (9)).

Annual Changes in the 5-Year Crude Survival Rate, Distribution of Clinical Stage, and Treatment for Breast Cancer Patients in Japan

During the 8-year period from 1963 to 1970, we observed no real variance in the 5-year crude survival and the recurrence-free survival rates. These respective rate averages stood at an annual 72.1% (based on a low of 68.5% and a high of 74.9% per annum) and 67.2% (low 64.8% and high 71.0%).

Viewed in terms of clinical stage treatment, we find the 4 basic stages reported as follows for 1963–1974:

Stage	Annual Average	Annual Rates
I	44%	(low) 40.5% (high) 48.5% per annum
II	30%	(low) 26.4% (high) 33.9% per annum

III   22.5%   (low) 18.0%   (high) 27.5% per annum

IV   3.5%   (low) 2.5%   (high) 4.9% per annum

For the reporting period (12 years), we again observe no real change in the distribution of percentages from year to year.

Regarding method of treatment during 1965–1974 surgery was in first place being employed in an annual average of 98.6% of all cases; hormonal therapy was the least employed methodology at an annual average 8.5%. Noteworthy, however, is the fact that radiotherapy fell from high use in 62.7% of all cases to a low of 26.6%. On the other hand, chemotherapy utilization rose from 27.7% to 49.6%.

The foregoing is based on reports from 38 major Japanese hospitals. Data from the Cancer Institute Hospital, however, is not included (Fujimori (8)).

Effect of Radiotherapy or Anticancer Agents in Combination with Surgery for Breast Cancer

Table I presents the crude survival rates of the total 1,793 breast cancer patients treated by the RGCTBC member during 1963–1965. The Table breaks down according to patients treated by surgery alone, as well as those treated by surgery in combination with postoperative radiotherapy and surgery with chemotherapy.

When viewed in terms of the total cases cared for by the three basic surgical procedures, i.e., typical radical mastectomy, modified radical mastectomy, and extended radical mastectomy, survival rates for patients receiving postoperative radiotherapy appear to be the lowest. This may be observed both in the total, as well as in the three separate surgical procedure columns in Table I. Accordingly, we are forced to assume that the value of radiotherapy (radium, cobalt 60 and linear accelerator) in postoperative treatment is low (Fujimori (8)).

TABLE I.   Ten-year Crude Survival Rate for Breast Cancer Treated during 1963–1965 Classified by Treatments

	Radical mastectomy	Modified radical mastectomy	Extended radical mastectomy	Total	
Surgery	79.8% (288/361)	66.4% (93/140)	54.4% (31/57)	74.2%	(412/558)
Surgery + radiotherpy	60.2% (490/814)	46.7% (21/45)	31.0% (58/187)	54.4%	(569/1,046)
Surgery + chemotherapy	64.2% (43/67)	71.4% (50/70)	57.7% (30/52)	65.1%	(123/189)
Total	66.1% (821/1,242)	64.3% (164/255)	40.2% (119/296)	61.6%	(1,104/1,793)
Significance of differences among three treatments (χ^2 test)	Highly significant ($p \ll 0.01$)	Significant ($0.010 < p < 0.025$)	Highly significant ($p \ll 0.005$)	Highly significant ($p \ll 0.01$)	

(Fujimori, M. et al. Research Group on "The Choice of Treatment for Breast Cancer" supported by the Ministry of Health and Welfare, 1976).

Relative Survival Rates for Breast Cancer Treated in Japan from 1960 to 1969

A total of 2,145 breast cancer cases treated during the period of 1960–1969 by the

TABLE II.   Relative Survival Rate for Breast Cancer Treated during 1960-1969

Period	LX	DX	UX	WX	L'X	QX	PX	P'X	E.S.R.	R.S.R.
0	2,145	2								
1	2,143	73	24	0	2,131.0	0.0343	0.9657	0.9657	0.9922	0.9734
2	2,046	137	13	0	2,039.5	0.0672	0.9328	0.9009	0.9838	0.9157
3	1,896	117	15	0	1,888.5	0.0620	0.9380	0.8451	0.9750	0.8667
4	1,764	104	12	0	1,758.0	0.0592	0.9408	0.7951	0.9656	0.8234
5	1,648	77	47	0	1,624.5	0.0474	0.9526	0.7574	0.9561	0.7922
6	1,524	68	323	2	1,361.5	0.0499	0.9501	0.7196	0.9455	0.7610
7	1,131	45	106	79	1,038.5	0.0433	0.9567	0.6884	0.9349	0.7363
8	901	33	112	70	810.0	0.0407	0.9593	0.6603	0.9235	0.7151
9	686	20	119	48	602.5	0.0332	0.9668	0.6384	0.9104	0.7013
10	499	17	22	44	466.0	0.0365	0.9635	0.6151	0.8967	0.6860

Period, year of observation; LX, alive at beginning of interval; DX, died during interval; UX, lost to follow-up during interval; WX, withdrawn alive during interval; L'X, effective number exposed to the risk of dying; QX, proportion dying; PX, proportion surviving; P'X, observed survival rate; E.S.R., expected survival rate; R.S.R., relative survival rate.

(Fujimori, M. *et al*. Research Group on " The Choice of Treatment for Breast Cancer " supported by Ministry of Health and Welfare, Japan, 1976).

RGCTBC member (Chairman M. Fujimori (8) with members H. Watanabe, O. Takatani, M. Yoshida, M. Izuo, T. Terasawa, S. Ikari, T. Seno, and T. Amaaki) were analyzed by making use of relative survival rate (R.S.R.) (Ederer (3)) computing method first adopted at the September 1963 "International Symposium on End Results of Cancer Therapy" (Norway). These results can be seen in Table II.

The 5-year R.S.R. was found to be 79.2%, and the 10-year R.S.R. was 68.6%. The percentage of cases lost to follow-up was 5.2% for the 5-year period, indicating that the 5-year R.S.R. data may be considered as highly reliable. On the other hand, cases lost to follow-up in the 10 year-category rose to over 10%, indicating that the 10-year R.S.R. data, as currently presented, are less reliable. However, we would note that it is still too early to render a true estimation of the final impact of cases withdrawn alive during the latter 5 years of the 10-year period.

Table III is classification of R.S.R. by clinical stage (TnM) and by surgical procedure.

> The "n" in TnM: The regional lymph node examined histologically (Japan Mammary Cancer Society (6)).
>
> Typical radical mastectomy (TRM): Radical mastectomy by the Halsted's, Meyer's, or Haagensen-Halsted's technique.
>
> Atypical radical mastectomy (ARM): Modified radical mastectomy (Patey's or Auchincloss's operation), or radical mastectomy without dissection of the minor pectoral muscles.
>
> Extended radical mastectomy (ERM): TRM with dissection of the parasternal or supraclavicular lymph nodes.
>
> Simple mastectomy (SM): Removal of mammary tissue (skin, subcutaneous tissue, and mammary gland). (RGCTBC (8)).

In the 5-year R.S.R. category, the ARM approach rates highest, TRM second, followed by ERM, when all four clinical stages are taken into calculation (see "Total"

TABLE III.   Relative Survival Rate for Breast Cancer Treated during 1960–1969
Classified by Clinical Stage and Surgical Procedure

Stage (TnM)	Relative survival	Radical mastectomy (cases)		Modified radical mastectomy (cases)		Extended radical mastectomy (cases)		Simple mastectomy (cases)		Total (cases)	
					Surgical procedure						
I	5-Year	0.9511	(587)	0.9763	(214)	0.9126	(203)	0.7925	(8)	0.9734	(1,012)
	10-Year	0.9115		0.9371		0.8704		0.6316		1.0622	
II	5-Year	0.7984	(341)	0.8641	(152)	0.8183	(170)	0.3368	(3)	0.8559	(666)
	10-Year	0.6055		0.8407		0.6627		—		0.7988	
III	5-Year	0.4506	(181)	0.4367	(41)	0.4905	(167)	—	(0)	0.4817	(389)
	10-Year	0.2297		0.3146		0.2553		—		0.2873	
IV	5-Year	0.2032	(26)	0.2513	(14)	0.1328	(36)	—	(2)	0.1782	(78)
	10-Year	0.1648		0.1816		0.0578		—		0.1400	
Total	5-Year	0.8090	(1,135)	0.8617	(421)	0.7146	(576)	0.5433	(13)	0.7922	(2,145)
	10-Year	0.6844		0.8195		0.5742		0.3438		0.6860	

(Fujimori, M. *et al.* Research Group on "The Choice of Treatment for Breast Cancer" supported by Ministry of Health and Welfare, Japan, 1976).

data in the "Stage" column). However, it is worth noting that there would appear to be no significant difference between the 5-year R.S.R. for the TRM, ARM, and the ERM approaches when viewed at each separate clinical stage.

In the 10-year R.S.R. category, we observe the same rating line-up for the ARM, TRM, and ERM approaches when all four clinical stages are considered. When observed by separate clinical stages (Stage I, III, and IV), no significant rating difference between the three approaches is seen. However, in clinical Stage II we find ARM rated higher than TRM. At this point, a statistical analysis, classified by histological types and by substages of TnM, was conducted for clinical Stage II breast cancer cases. The results would appear to verify the 10-year R.S.R. differences shown in Table III. However, in evaluating these data, we would suggest that the lower reliability for the 10-year R.S.R. figures referred to earlier in this appear be taken into account.

Table IV is a comparison, based upon the computational methods noted previously, of R.S.R. for breast cancer treatment in Japan, Norway, and U.S.A. At the reliable 5-year R.S.R., it is found that R.S.R. in Japan stands at 79.2% against 65% in Norway and 63% in U.S.A. (Cutler (*1*, *2*)).

Figure 1 relates the histological types of breast cancer to the four basic clinical stages. Therein, non-infiltrating carcinoma is rated highest in Stage I, with scirrhous carcinoma being most prevalent in Stage II, III, and IV. A markedly similar break-

TABLE IV.   Relative Survival Rates for Breast Cancer, An International Comparison

Country	No. of cases	5-Year R.S.R. (%)	10-Year R.S.R. (%)
U.S.A.	15,653	63	50
Norway	879	65	49
Japan	2,145	79.2	68.6

Breast cancer, all types and all stages.

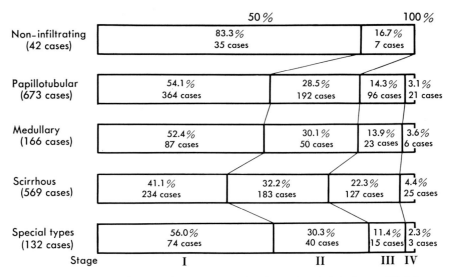

FIG. 1.   Histological types of breast cancer (1960–1969) and their Stages (TnM)
(Fujimori, M. *et al.* Research Group on "The Choice of Treatment for Breast
Cancer" supported by Japanese Ministry of Health and Welfare, 1976).

TABLE V.   Relative Survival Rates for Each Histological Type of Breast Cancer,
Comparison between Norway and Japan[a]

Norway			Japan		
	5-Year R.S.R. (%)	10-Year R.S.R. (%)		5-Year R.S.R. (%)	10-Year R.S.R. (%)
All types	65	49	All types	79.2	68.5
Medullary type	64	43	Medullary type	84.6	75.0
Papillary type	31	31	Papillotubular type	82.9	74.1
Comedo carcinoma	67	46	Scirrhous type	73.2	60.3
Nonspecific type	64	49	Other types[b]	87.9	79.9
Mucinous type	87	92			

[a] Histological classifications used in Norway and Japan were not identical, but some types are found
to be comparable.

[b] Other types include lobular carcinoma, mucinous carcinoma, apocrine type carcinoma, and other
specific types.

down for papillotubular carcinoma and for medullary carcinoma may be observed in
Fig. 1.

Table V compares R.S.R. by histological type of breast cancer treatment in Japan
(Fujimori (*8*)) and Norway (Cutler (*1*)). In this Table, we note that the Japan R.S.R.
is the highest in all cases.

Recurrence of Breast Cancer after Surgical Treatment

Viewed in terms of the rate of local recurrence of 2,335 breast cancer cases within
10 years after radical mastectomy during the period of 1960–1969 by 7 members

TABLE VI. Local Recurrence of Breast Cancer within 10 Years
after Radical Mastectomy during 1960-1969

Stage (TnM)	Recurrence			
	Site and percentage of recurrence (No. of recurrence/No. of mastectomy)			
	Chest wall	Parasternum	Axilla	Total
I	2.9% (36/1,235)	0.6% (8/1,235)	0.2% (2/1,235)	3.7% (46/1,235)
II	4.6% (30/643)	0.8% (5/643)	0 % (0/643)	5.4% (35/643)
III	14.1% (56/396)	1.0% (4/396)	0.8% (3/396)	15.9% (63/396)
IV	14.8% (9/61)	0 % (0/61)	0 % (0/61)	14.8% (9/61)
Total	5.6% (131/2,335)	0.7% (17/2,335)	0.2% (5/2,335)	6.5% (153/2,335)

Cases lost to follow-up (159 cases) are excluded from this Table.

Percentage of cases lost to follow-up is 6.3%.

Chest wall denotes the local site around the scar of surgery.

(Fujimori, M. Research Group on " The Choice of Treatment for Breast Cancer " supported by the Ministry of Health and Welfare, 1976).

TABLE VII. Recurrence of Breast Cancer (1965-1971) of Stage I (UICC) in Japan

	No. of cases	No. of recurrence	Percentage of recurrence
$T_1N_0M_0$	1,894	111	5.9
$T_2N_0M_0$	2,543	282	11.1
Stage I	4,437[a]	393	8.9

[a] The number of cases of Stage I: 4,437 accounts for 37.9% of the total number of cases: 11,708.
(Fujimori, M. Japan Mammary Cancer Society, 1972).

of the RGCTBC, we find an overall rate of 6.5% (Stage I, 3.7%; Stage II, 5.4%; Stage III, 15.9%; Stage IV, 14.8%); and the chest wall is the most frequent site of local recurrences (Table VI).

Further, when viewed in terms of the rate and site of all recurrences (local and distant) of Stage I breast cancer cases treated during 1965–1971 by members of the Japan Mammary Cancer Society, the rate stands at 8.9% and the hematogen metastasis is responsible for about 60% of all cases (Tables VII and VIII) (Fujimori (8)).

Radiotherapy, Chemotherapy, and Hormonal Therapy for Breast Cancer

Radiotherapy has been employed for several decades in Japan in the treatment of breast cancer. Numerous new approaches in this field are now in existence, but viewed historically, X-ray and radium (2,000–2,500 rad) were first used. X-ray was then followed by cobalt 60 (about 5,000 rad), with linear accelerator (5,000–6,000 rad) and Betatron therapy appearing in recent years. Those employing radiotherapy in the preoperative stage here are in the minority, with the majority using radiation as postoperative therapy. Despite the disappointing results noted in Table I, hopes are held for the future of radiotherapy in the treatment of breast cancer.

The use of anticancer agents in chemotherapy has been increasing since the latter half of the 1960's. Here in Japan the leading agents employed in the treatment of

TABLE VIII. Recurrence of Breast Cancer (1965–1971) of Stage I (UICC) in Japan

Site and percentage of recurrence	Stage					
	T_1		T_2		T_1+T_2 (Stage I)	
	n_0[a]	Total	n_0[a]	Total	n_0[a]	Total
	71[b]	109[b]	133[b]	255[b]	204[b]	364[b]
Lung	25.4	25.7	23.3	22.7	24.0	23.6
Bone	22.5	21.1	19.5	19.2	20.5	19.5
Local skin	11.3	19.3	23.3	16.1	19.1	17.0
Regional lymph node	16.9	18.3	15.0	13.3	15.7	14.8
Liver	4.2	4.6	12.8	13.3	9.8	10.7
Pleura	8.5	8.3	3.0	6.3	4.9	6.9
Distant lymph node	11.3	7.3	3.0	5.9	5.8	6.3
Contralateral breast	1.4	0.9	6.0	6.7	4.4	4.9
Peritoneum	4.2	3.7	—	0.8	1.5	1.6
Brain	1.4	0.9	3.0	2.0	1.5	1.6
Distant skin	2.8	1.8	0.8	1.2	1.5	1.4
Ovary	1.4	0.9	3.0	1.6	1.5	1.4
Pericardium	1.4	0.9	—	0.4	—	0.3
Uterus	—	—	—	0.4	—	0.3

[a] n_0 denotes the negative involvement histologically of axillary lymph nodes.
(Fujimori, M. Japan Mammary Cancer Society, 1972).
[b] Cases of recurrence.

TABLE IX. Effect of Anticancer Agents for Advanced Breast Cancer (1965–1974)

Anticancer agents	No. of cases	Objective improvement for more than 6 months (%)
Cyclophosphamide (100–200 mg, p.o., per day)	184	39
Mitomycin C (4 mg, p.o., per day, 4 weeks)	76	25
5-Fluorouracil (300 mg, p.o., per day)	53	34
Combination of multiple drugs[a]	96	47

[a] Cyclophosphamide (50 mg), mitomycin C (2 mg), 5-fluorouracil (100 mg), and prednisone (10 mg) are given per day.
(Fujimori, M. et al. Research Group on " The Choice of Treatment for Breast Cancer " supported by the Ministry of Health and Welfare, 1975).

breast cancer are cyclophosphamide, mitomycin C, and 5-fluorouracil. In the early years the tendency was toward separate administration of these agents in the treatment of advanced breast cancer. Recently, however, the trend has been toward a combined administration of multiple drugs. As may be seen in Table IX, objective improvement for more than 6 months in advanced breast cancer cases appears to be best obtained through combined administration of anticancer agents (Fujimori (8)).

I have conducted regional perfusion of mitomycin C as adjuvant therapy for breast cancer, and am conducting a continuing investigation of the 5-year crude survival rate. Table X presents the data obtained to date; results, unfortunately, remain inconclusive (Fujimori (4)).

Significant employment of hormonal therapy for advanced breast cancer began

TABLE X. Effect of Regional Perfusion of MMC as Adjuvant Chemotherapy
for Breast Cancer (1964–1969)

Stage (TNM)	5-Year survival rate	
	Radical mastectomy	Radical mastectomy with regional perfusion
I	86.5% (45/52)	95.0% (19/20)
II	89.8% (44/49)	81.1% (30/37)
III	68.2% (15/22)	80.0% (16/20)
Total	84.5% (104/123)	84.4% (65/77)

Difference in 5-year survival rates between radical mastectomy and radical mastectomy with regional perfusion is not significant by χ^2 test or test for difference of proportion.
(Fujimori, M., 1973).

TABLE XI. Effect of Hormone Therapies for Advanced Breast Cancer (1965–1974) in Japan

Treatment	Number of cases	Improvement (%)	Average period of remission in improved cases (months)
Therapeutic oophorectomy	107	16.8	23.4
Adrenalectomy after oophorectomy	23	34.8	13.7
Adrenalectomy with oophorectomy	22	36.4	30.6
Holotestine (20 mg per day)	73	17.8	14.6
Diethylstilbestrol (50 mg per day)	43	25.6	14.6

(Fujimori, M. et al. Research Group on "The Choice of Treatment for Breast Cancer" supported by the Ministry of Health and Welfare, 1974).

TABLE XII. Effect of Therapeutic Oophorectomy for Breast Cancer

Authors	Year	No. of cases	Objective regression (%)	Remarks
Treves	1954	156	44.0	Premenopausal
Treves	1954		22.0	Postmenopausal
Pearson	1955	75	44.0	Premenopausal
Pearson	1955	21	10.0	Postmenopausal
Dao	1962	84	32.0	Premenopausal
Taylor	1962	381	29.7	Joint Committee
Kennedy	1964	177	47.5	
Fujimori	1971	315[a]	28.6	Japan Mammary Cancer Society Regression >6 months

[a] Cases treated from 1965 to 1969.

at least as early as the 1950's. From that time, to the present, therapeutic oophorectomy, adrenalectomy after or with oophorectomy, and the administration of Halotestine or diethylstilbestrol have been employed.

We would note, however, that the use of hormonal therapy appears to have stabilized at less than 10% of the breast cancer cases reported in Japan. As may be observed in Tables XI, XII, and XIII, dealing with the effects of hormonal therapy,

TABLE XIII.   Effect of Adrenalectomy for Breast Cancer

Authors	Year	No. of cases	Objective regression (%)	Remarks
Fracchia	1959	155	43.0	
Hellström	1959	233	42.0	
Daicoff	1962	455	28.0	Regression>6 months
Byron	1962	248	37.7	
McDonald	1962	690	28.4	Joint Committee Regression>6 months
Prohaska	1965	566	28.0	
Tonemoto and Byron	1967	340	32.0	
Fracchia	1967	500	35.6	Regression>6 months
Fujimori	1971	443[a]	27.5	Japan Mammary Cancer Society Regression>6 months

[a] Cases treated during 1965–1969.

the average period of remission stands at 15 to 30%, adrenalectomy with oophorectomy appearing to have had the best results (Fujimori (7, 8)).

In conclusion we note that in recent years we have started research on an estrogen receptor as an indicator for hormonal therapy.

Acknowledgments

I am indebted to members of the research group on "The Choice of Treatments for Breast Cancer" supported by the Japanese Ministry of Health and Welfare, K. Kuno (Cancer Institute), H. Kaneda (Cancer Institute), H. Watanabe (St. Marianna University School of Medicine), O. Takatani (National Cancer Center), M. Izuo (Gunma University School of Medicine), T. Terasawa (Center for Adult Disease, Osaka), M. Yoshida (Aichi Cancer Center), T. Amaaki (Keio University), T. Seno (Kawasaki Medical College), S. Ikari (Tachikawa Kyosai Hospital), R. Usui (Takasaki National Hospital) as co-workers of this study. I am also grateful to Drs. T. Kubo, Y. Higashi, and Mr. T. Tanaka (Saitama Cancer Center) for their help in the statistical work.

REFERENCES

1.   Cutler, S. J., Black, M. M., Mork, T., Harvei, S., and Freeman, C. Further observations on prognostic factors in cancer of the female breast. *Cancer*, **24**, 653–667 (1969).
2.   Cutler, S. J. and Heise, H. W. Long-term end results of treatment of cancer. *J. Am. Med. Assoc.*, **216**, 293–297 (1971).
3.   Ederer, F., Axtell, L. M., and Cutler, S. J. The relative survival rate: A statistical methodology. *Natl. Cancer Inst. Monogr.*, **6**, 101–121 (1961).
4.   Fujimori, M., Sakauchi, G., Izuo, M., Abe, C., Morita, S., Nashimoto, T., Ishikawa, S., Sadamitsu, H., and Kawai, T. Studies on regional perfusion and intra-arterial infusion for cancer chemotherapy. *Surgery*, **55**, 630–639 (1964).
5.   Fujimori, M. Postoperative prognosis of breast cancer. *In* "The Year Book of Cancer," ed. by Clark et Cumley, Year Book Medical Publishers, Chicago, pp. 95–96 (1970).
6.   Fujimori, M. General rules for clinical and histological record of mammary cancer. *Japan. J. Surg.*, **5**, 118–131 (1975).
7.   Fujimori, M. Surgical hormone therapy for breast cancer. *Nippon Gan Chiryo Gakkai-shi* (*J. Japan. Soc. Cancer Ther.*), **7**, 56–63 (1972) (in Japanese).

8. Fujimori, M. Studies on the choice of treatments for breast cancer. *Kosei-sho Gan Kenkyu Hokoku-shu* (*Annu. Rep. Cancer Res. Ministry Health and Welfare*), 65–73 (1971).
9. Hirayama, T. Epidemiology of Cancer. *Rep. Japan Union, Cancer*, **73**, 1–8 (1973) (in Japanese).
10. Kajitani, T. Breast Cancer. *Nippon Geka Zensho* (*Japan. Comp. Surg.*), **14**, 303–424 (1957) (in Japanese).

CANCER OF THE BREAST AT
CANCER INSTITUTE HOSPITAL, TOKYO

Keijiro Kuno and Atsuo Fukami

*Cancer Institute Hospital**

The 5-year relative survival rate of 1,386 primary cases of breast carcinoma operated in the Cancer Institute Hospital from 1960 to 1970 was 79.6%, and the 10-year relative survival rate of 652 cases operated on from 1960 to 1965 was 66.1%. The 5-year relative survival rates according to the TNM staging were 90.1% for Stage I, 79.9% for Stage II, and 47.1% for Stage III; the 10-year relative survival rates were 81.0% for Stage I, 67.1% for Stage II, and 22.7% for Stage III. The number of metastasized axillary lymph nodes had the strongest effect on the prognosis of breast carcinoma. It had been the custom to carry out standard radical mastectomy for the majority of cases, but modified radical mastectomy is now being carried out for Stage I cases.

According to Segi's statistics (6), the age-adjusted death rates from breast carcinoma in Japanese females is 3.80 per 100,000 female population; this is the lowest among 24 countries listed. The reason for the small incidence of breast carcinoma in Japanese females is still not clear, even from epidemiological investigations. However, the number of breast carcinoma patients has been showing a tendency to increase in Japan during the past few years.

In the Department of Surgery, Cancer Institute Hospital, Tokyo, a total of 2,789 primary cases of breast carcinoma in females were operated on during 1946–1974. The age of breast carcinoma patients shows a peak at 45–49 years, comprising 21.0% of the whole, followed by those aged 40–44 years (18.9%) and those of 50–54 years (14.7%) (Fig. 1). The youngest patient was aged 21 and the oldest was 89, with an

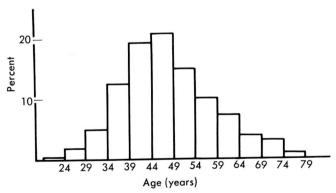

Fig. 1. Age distribution of 2,789 patients with breast cancer (1960–1970, Cancer Institute Hospital, Tokyo)

* Kami-Ikebukuro 1-37-1, Toshima-ku, Tokyo 170, Japan (久野敬二郎, 深見敦夫).

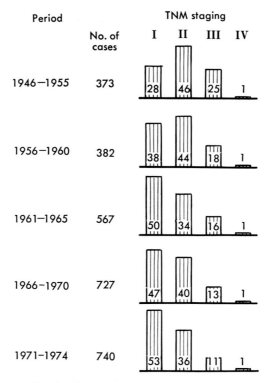

FIG. 2.   TNM staging by 5-year periods

average age of 48 years. This average age is 4–5 years younger than that of breast carcinoma patients in Europe and the U.S.A.

The TNM staging (UICC, 1968) of the primary cases operated on during 1946–1974 was 45.2% of Stage I, 38.8% of Stage II, 15.4% of Stage III, and 0.6% of Stage IV. The small number of Stage IV cases means that they were treated by radiation and not by surgery. As shown in Fig. 2, the rate of early carcinoma of the breast has been increasing gradually.

The 5-year crude survival rate is shown in Fig. 3 according to stages, and comparison of the figures for 1946–1955 with those for 1966–1969 shows only a 10% increase in the 5-year survival rate of cases in Stage III.

End Results

The 5-year end results of 1,386 primary cases of breast carcinoma operated on during 1960–1970 consisted of 1,076 cases surviving for 5 years and 310 cases of death, among which 207 cases died from recurrence, 101 cases from intercurrent or unknown disease, and 2 cases as a direct result of surgery. There were no cases lost to follow-up. The 5-year crude survival rate is 77.6%, the 5-year relative survival rate calculated from the life table is 79.6%.

The 10-year end results of 652 cases operated on during 1960–1965 consisted of 412 cases who lived for 10 years and 240 cases who died, including 149 cases from

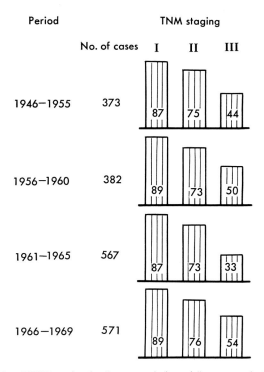

FIG. 3.   TNM staging by 5-year periods and 5-year survival rate

recurrence, 90 cases from intercurrent or unknown disease, and one case as a direct result of surgery. There were no cases lost to follow-up. The 10-year crude survival rate is 63.2% and the 10-year relative survival rate is 66.1%.

TNM Staging

Prognosis of breast carcinoma cases according to TNM staging, excluding simultaneous bilateral breast carcinoma and direct death from surgery, is shown in Table I. The 5-year relative survival rate was 90.1% for 660 cases of Stage I, 79.9% for 521 cases of Stage II, 47.1% for 195 cases of Stage III, and 0% for 4 cases of Stage IV. The 10-year relative survival rate was 81.0% for 314 cases of Stage I, 67.1% for 229 cases of Stage II, 22.7% for 100 cases of Stage III, and 0% for 2 cases of Stage IV.

TABLE I.   TNM Staging and Relative Survival Rate

TNM stage	5-Year survival		10-Year survival	
	No.	%	No.	%
I	660	90.1	314	81.0
II	521	79.9	229	67.1
III	195	47.1	100	22.7
IV	4	0	2	0

Treatment

In the Cancer Institute Hospital, Tokyo, Halsted standard radical mastectomy is carried out on majority of cases with breast carcinoma and modified radical mastectomy for the very early carcinoma cases. For some of the advanced cases, parasternal dissection or supraclavicular dissection or extended radical mastectomy for dissection of both is carried out. In the standard radical mastectomy, the skin flap is thin, the pars costalis of the pectoralis major muscle and pectoralis minor muscle are dissected, and axillar and subclavicular lymph nodes are thoroughly dissected. To overcome the skin defect, a skin graft is carried out in 80% of the cases. Among 1,151 cases given standard radical mastectomy, the 5-year relative survival rate was 85.9% and 10-year relative survival rate was 70.1% (Table II).

In modified radical mastectomy, Patey's operation (5), retaining the pectoral major and dissecting the pectoral minor, or Auchincloss operation (1), retaining both pectoral muscles, has been carried out on about half of the breast carcinoma patients in recent years, although the previous surgery was to dissect the pectoral major and retain the pectoral minor. The 5-year relative survival rate in 41 cases given modified radical mastectomy was 76.8% and the 10-year relative survival rate was 65.0%.

The 5-year relative survival rate was 56.6% for 174 cases given extended radical mastectomy during 1960–1970, including 85 cases of parasternal dissection, 50 cases of supraclavicular dissection, and 39 cases of parasternal and supraclavicular dissection. The 10-year relative survival rate was 28.7% in 51 cases given extended radical mastectomy during 1960–1965, including 22 cases of parasternal dissection, 24 cases of supraclavicular dissection, and 5 cases of parasternal and supraclavicular dissection. Extended radical mastectomy cannot improve the prognosis and radiotherapy is now being used.

Postoperative irradiation was made with ^{137}Cs distant irradiation during 1960–1963, with ^{60}Co from 1963, and from 1966, the Linac accelerator has been used to give an irradiation dose of 5,000 R over 4 weeks to the supra- and infra-clavicular region and parasternal region. On principle, local and axillar irradiation is not given. Postoperative irradiation is carried out routinely for cases with positive axillary metastasis but not in early carcinoma, so that a comparison of prognosis between these groups cannot be made.

As postoperative chemotherapy, short-period administration of 0.6–0.8 mg/kg of mitomycin-C was made in 178 cases during 1968–1970, but there was no significant difference in the survival rate between this group and the nonadministered group.

TABLE II. Type of Mastectomy and Relative Survival Rate

Type of mastectomy	5-Year survival		10-Year survival	
	No.	%	No.	%
Standard radical mastectomy	1,151	85.9	567	70.1
Modified radical mastectomy	41	76.8	24	65.0
Extended radical mastectomy	174	56.6	51	28.7

Size of Tumor

Relation between the longer diameter of the primary cancer, measured on surgical specimens, and the 5-year relative survival rate is shown in Table III. The 5-year survival was 95.6% in 141 cases with a tumor less than 1.0 cm, 91.1% in 463 cases with a tumor size of 1.1–2.0 cm, 82.0% in 364 cases with a tumor of 2.1–3.0 cm, 68.0% in 196 cases with a tumor size of 3.1–4.0 cm, 66.1% in 90 cases with a tumor size of 4.1–5.0 cm, and 50.4% in 108 cases with a tumor size of over 5.1 cm, showing that prognosis becomes poorer as the tumor size increases.

TABLE III. Size of Tumor and Relative Survival Rate

Size of tumor (cm)	5-Year survival		10-Year survival	
	No.	%	No.	%
−1.0	141	95.6	65	90.8
1.1–2.0	463	91.1	229	82.9
2.1–3.0	364	82.0	174	59.3
3.1–4.0	196	68.0	90	45.4
4.1–5.0	90	66.1	39	43.3
5.1–	108	50.4	44	30.8

Axillary Metastasis

Metastasis to the axillary lymph nodes is a factor that most affects prognosis. The 5-year relative survival rate according to the number of histologically confirmed metastasized lymph nodes was 95.0% in 709 cases without metastasis, 80.4% in 354 cases with 1–3 nodes involved, 51.3% in 165 cases with 4–9 nodes involved, and 39.0% in 136 cases with more than 10 nodes involved. The 10-year relative survival rate was 87.9% in 335 cases without metastasis, 62.2% in 165 cases with 1–3 nodes involved, 27.3% in 81 cases with 4–9 nodes involved, and 13.0% in 58 cases with more than 10 nodes involved (Table IV).

TABLE IV. Axillary Metastases and Relative Survival Rate

No. of positive nodes	5-Year survival		10-Year survival	
	No.	%	No.	%
0	709	95.0	355	87.9
1–3	354	80.4	165	62.2
4–9	165	51.3	81	27.3
10–	136	39.0	58	13.0

Histological Classification

There are many kinds of pathological classification of breast cancer and we use the histological classification established by the Japan Mammary Cancer Society (4). The infiltrating carcinoma is divided into the common type and special type. There are no recurrences in the noninfiltrating carcinoma. The relationship between the

TABLE V. Histological Types and Relative Survival Rate

Histological type	5-Year survival		10-Year survival	
	No.	%	No.	%
Noninfiltrating carcinoma	45	93.9	29	87.2
Infiltrating carcinoma				
Common type				
Papillotubular carcinoma	269	88.5	149	75.7
Medullary tubular carcinoma	300	77.8	87	64.3
Scirrhous carcinoma	657	76.9	331	60.4
Special type	97	84.9	50	83.7

histological classification of breast carcinoma and 5- and 10-year relative survival rates is listed in Table V.

Tnm Staging

In some cases, clinical judgement of axillary lymph node(s) before surgery does not agree with postoperative histological findings. Histological metastasis was found in 25% of N_0 and 38% of N_{1a}, but in 14% of N_{1b}, there was no histological metastasis. The degree of metastasis found by histological examination of the lymph nodes is classified as n_0, n_1, n_2, and n_3 by the Japan Mammary Cancer Society, and a Tnm classification was established by combination with T from TNM staging (Fig. 4).

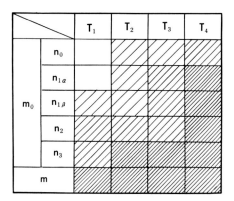

FIG. 4. Stage grouping in TNM classification
☐ Stage I; ▨ Stage II; ▨ Stage III; ▨ Stage IV.

TABLE VI. Tnm Staging and Relative Survival Rate

Tnm stage	5-Year survival		10-Year survival	
	No.	%	No.	%
I	763	94.0	375	88.5
II	336	76.9	128	52.7
III	220	48.0	129	21.8
IV	40	39.1	13	8.3

Tnm classification expresses the progress of breast carcinoma better than the TNM staging based on clinical judgement.

The 5-year relative survival rates according to Tnm staging were 94.0% for 763 cases of Stage I, 76.9% of 336 cases of Stage II, 48.0% for 220 cases of Stage III, and 39.1% for 40 cases of Stage IV. The 10-year survival rates were 88.5% for 375 cases of Stage I, 52.7% for 128 cases of Stage II, 21.8% for 129 cases of Stage III, and 8.3% for 13 cases of Stage IV.

CONCLUSIONS

In spite of many clinical trials, surgical treatment and adjuvant therapy have not been established as the proper primary treatment for breast carcinoma. In the majority of breast cancer cases, standard radical mastectomy has been carried out but, because of an increase in Stage I cases in recent years, modified radical mastectomy has been carried out for such cases, and the results are being examined by a careful follow-up.

Japanese women have smaller breasts than women in Europe and America. This means that Japanese women are more likely to discover a tumorous mass earlier. The smaller breast size is advantageous for clinical palpation but disadvantageous for judging the tumor shadow in mammography. About one-half of the carcinomata being treated at present are less than 2 cm in diameter. This is one of the reasons that the result of treatment of breast carcinoma in Japan is better than in European and American countries. Even with the same size of tumor, prognosis is better in Japan. It has been said that there must be a factor that makes breast carcinoma less frequent in Japan and that this factor allows a better prognosis, but this factor has not been clarified. The endocrine environment may be responsible for the difference in the incidence of breast carcinoma between Japan and other countries.

REFERENCES

1. Auchincloss, H. Significance of location and number of axillary metastases in carcinoma of the breast; a justification for a conservative operation. *Ann. Surg.*, **158**, 37–46 (1963).
2. Fisher, B., Slack, N. H., Bross, and I.D.J. Cancer of the breast: Size of neoplasm and prognosis. *Cancer*, **24**, 1071–1080 (1969).
3. Fisher, B. Cooperative clinical trials in primary breast cancer: A critical appraisal. *Cancer*, **31**, 1271–1286 (1973).
4. Japan Mammary Cancer Society. General rules for clinical and histological recording of mammary cancer. *Japan. J. Surg.*, **5**, 118–131, 175–185 (1975).
5. Patey, D. H. A review of 146 cases of the breast operated on between 1930 and 1943. *Br. J. Cancer*, **21**, 260–269 (1967).
6. Segi, M., Kurihara, M., and Matsuyama, T. "Cancer Mortality for Selected Sites in 24 Countries" No. 5, 1964–1965. Dept. Public Health, Tohoku University School of Medicine, Sendai (1969).
7. Wynder, E. R., Kajitani, T., Kuno, K., Lucas, J. C., Pals, A. D., and Farrow, J. A comparison of survival rates between American and Japanese patients with breast cancer. *Surg. Gynecol. Obstet.*, **117**, 196–200 (1963).

OSTEOSARCOMA: INTRA-ARTERIAL INFUSION CHEMOTHERAPY COMBINED WITH SURGERY

Isao AOIKE,[*1] Yoshihiko AKAHOSHI,[*2] and Hisatoshi FUKUMA[*3]

*Department of Orthopaedic Surgery, Tokyo Medical and Dental University,[*1]
Department of Orthopaedic Surgery, Gifu University Medical School,[*2] and
Department of Orthopaedic Surgery, National Cancer Center Hospital[*3]*

Since 1963, regional intra-arterial infusion of anticancer agents combined with surgery has been used in the treatment of osteosarcoma. This regimen is widely adopted at present in Japan in approximately half of the 45 institutions to which a questionnaire about the method of treatment of osteosarcoma was sent.

Through the histological examination of the limbs receiving intra-arterial infusion therapy, remarkable degeneration and necrosis were demonstrated throughout the area of the tumor tissue.

In the initial 2 weeks of infusion therapy local effects such as reduction of pain, decrease in local temperature, and regression of tumor size, as well as systemic effects such as decrease in the alkaline phosphatase level and in the erythrocyte sedimentation rate, were observed.

The 5-year survivors number 21 out of 53 cases which were followed for more than 5 years. The relative 5-year survival rate of this series was 42.9%. In this series 15 cases who underwent initial radical excision were included.

The management of patients with osteosarcoma is one of the most difficult tasks of the orthopedic surgeon. Surgical ablation is usually carried out at an early stage, but the results have not been satisfactory.

In 1956, the Japanese Orthopaedic Association started to record bone tumor cases, and since 1964 the National Cancer Center has published an annual report (*15*) concerning the incidence of bone tumors in Japan. During 1964–1974, 18,136 cases of bone tumors were reported, and of these, 2,031 (11.2%) were primary malignant tumors of the bone and 1,198 (6.6%) were osteosarcomas.

The more than 3-year survival rates of primary malignant bone tumors registered in 1972 are as follows: 29.5% of 93 osteosarcomas, 83.3% of 6 parosteal osteosarcomas, 48.1% of 27 chondrosarcomas, 63.6% of 11 fibrosarcomas, 37.5% of reticulum cell sarcomas, and 9.0% of Ewing's sarcomas (*15*).

Two hundred and eighty-seven cases of osteosarcoma treated until 1956 were analyzed in 1961 and 14.3% had survived more than 5 years. Eighty-seven patients had early amputation within 2 months after the onset of disease and 46 of these died

[*1] Yushima 1-5-45, Bunkyo-ku, Tokyo 113, Japan (青池勇雄).
[*2] Tsukasa-cho 40, Gifu 500, Japan (赤星義彦).
[*3] Tsukiji 5-1-1, Chuo-ku, Tokyo 104, Japan (福間久俊).

within one year, 27 within 3 years, 3 within 5 years, and the rest (only 8 patients) remained alive for more than 5 years (3).

Hematogenous pulmonary metastases may be present at an early stage of the disease in many of the cases but these could not be detected radiologically for several months after the onset of metastases.

The treatment of osteosarcoma in the past consisted of surgical ablation with the hope that pulmonary micrometastasis had not occurred. However, most patients died within 2 years due to pulmonary metastasis (10).

The development of pulmonary metastasis is the most important factor in determining the survival rate in patients with osteosarcoma. The surgical removal of the tumor prior to the occurrence of metastasis is the ideal treatment of this disease. Unfortunately, it is very difficult to detect osteosarcomas clinically before pulmonary metastasis has occurred. In most cases, the tumor has already invaded or widely destroyed the bone, and micrometastasis has occurred by the time a definitive diagnosis can be attained (1).

Adjuvant therapy should be given to prevent pulmonary metastasis and slow down the progression of the existing lesion. Radiotherapy, chemotherapy, and immunotherapy have been developed and applied in order to improve the rate of cure.

Osteosarcoma has been considered a radioresistant and chemotherapeutic-resistant tumor but, recent experience with new agents and administration of older agents in different dosages and schedules have proved to be efficient for the treatment of osteosarcoma.

The administration of chemotherapeutic agents is classified into three different types: Systemic intravenous administration, isolation intra-arterial perfusion, and regional intra-arterial infusion.

An inquiry was made of 45 Japanese institutions for the treatment of osteosarcomas; 86% of these institutions were using adjuvant therapy and half of these were using the specific infusion chemotherapy.

The method of specific infusion chemotherapy was first introduced by Klopp (7) in 1950, but it became popular in Japan after Akahoshi (2) reported good results in the treatment of osteosarcoma of the limbs (1967).

The present paper shows the analysis and clinical results of 53 cases of osteosarcoma; 35 from the Department of Orthopaedic Surgery at Gifu University, 11 from the Department of Orthopaedic Surgery at Tokyo Medical and Dental University, and 7 from the National Cancer Center Hospital. For proper evaluation of the treatment, parosteal osteosarcoma, radiation-induced sarcoma, and those of the pagetoid bone were excluded from this study.

Portable Chronometric Infusor

For regional intra-arterial infusion chemotherapy, the finest Teflon catheter and a portable chronometric infusor, which consisted of small pump, were used (Fig. 1).

Using a small infusor presented various advantages such as giving a more favorable mental effect on a patient and securing safer and longer infusion without the danger of infection which a large pump may have caused, and it would have needed an irrigator and syringe.

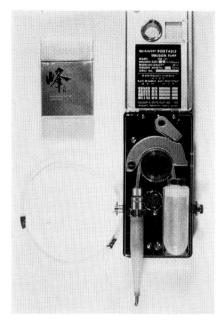

FIG. 1. Inner aspect of portable chronometric infusor with the Teflon catheter
Cigarette case (left, top) for comparing the size
Solution of drugs is infused at the rate of 5 ml per 24 hr from the drug reservoir
(20 ml).

Attention was paid to prevent complications and to lessen the systemic intoxication especially when the infusion was given continuously for a long period.

Technique of Insertion

In general, the Teflon catheter was inserted retrogradely into a branch of the main artery and was fixed. Intra-arterial infusion following amputation or wide resection was carried out very carefully in order to prevent injury of the peripheral tissues and the inner wall of the artery. The tip of the catheter was fixed finely in order to infuse an exact amount of the anticancer agents in the right place. The fluorescin method was used in order to confirm the infused area.

The anticancer agents used in most cases were mitomycin C (8–12 mg, twice a week), adriamycin (0.6 mg/kg, 3 days), 5-fluorouracil (1,000–15,000 mg/week) and methotrexate (100–150 mg/week). Two of these agents were infused simultaneously.

Regional intra-arterial infusion of the anticancer agents was started when the biopsy was made and it was continued for 3 to 6 weeks; radical ablation was then performed when the condition of the patient was good.

In a few cases simultaneous intra-arterial infusion and irradiation using ^{60}Co were carried out. Systemic chemotherapy was routinely used postoperatively. Bronchial arterial infusion was performed postoperatively in some patients at 3-month intervals.

Results

Histologically, tumor tissue obtained from amputated limbs treated by continuous intra-arterial infusion showed marked pycnosis and karyolysis throughout wide areas. In some cases no viable tumor cells could be found.

Clinically, the local effects of intra-arterial infusion during the initial 2 weeks of therapy included a reduction of pain, a decrease in local temperature, and regression of the tumor size. A decrease in the alkaline phosphatase level and in the erythrocyte sedimentation rate was also observed during the period of infusion (Fig. 2).

The age of the patients in this series ranged from 8 to 42 years at the time of diagnosis. The median age was 16.2 years. Twenty-nine of the patients were males and 24 females.

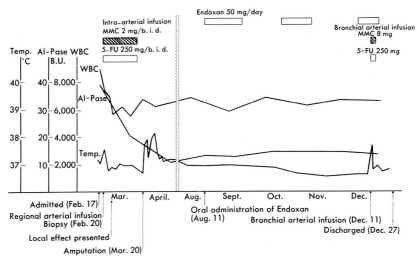

Y. K. 10 years ♀ Osteosarcoma of lt. femur

FIG. 2. Clinical course of osteosarcoma after intra-arterial infusion chemotherapy

MMC, mitomycin C; 5-FU, 5-fluorouracil; Al-Pase, alkalinephosphatase.

TABLE I.   Computation of Relative 5-Year Survival Rates

$x \sim x+1$	Lx	Dx	Ux	Wx	L'x Lx−1/2 (Nx+Wx)	Qx Dx/L'x	px (1−Qx)	Px P₁P₂P₃ ...Px	Expected rates (%)	Relative rates (%)
0–1	53	12	—	—	53	0.226	0.774	0.774	99.9	77.4
1–2	41	9	—	—	41	0.219	0.781	0.604	99.8	60.5
2–3	32	5	—	—	32	0.156	0.844	0.508	99.7	50.9
3–4	26	2	—	1	25.5	0.078	0.922	0.418	99.6	46.9
4–5	23	2	—	1	22.5	0.088	0.912	0.427	99.5	42.9
5–6	21				21					

$x \sim x+1$, year of observation; Lx, alive at beginning of interval; Dx, died during interval; Ux, lost to follow-up during interval; Wx, withdrawn alive during interval; L'x, effective number exposed to the risk of dying; Qx, proportion dying; px, proportion surviving; Px, cumulative proportion surviving.

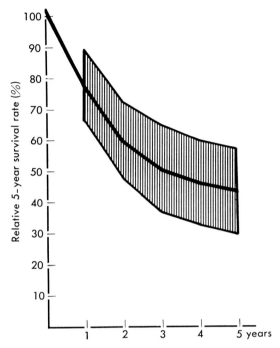

FIG. 3.   Computation of relative 5-year survival rates

Twelve patients died within 1 year and 21 of 53 patients survived longer than 5 years. The mortality within the first year was 22.6% and the relative 1-year survival rate was 77.4% (Table I). The relative 5-year survival rate (8) was 42.9% with a 95% confidence limit (±two standard deviation 13.6%) of 29.3% to 56.5% (Fig. 3). Fifteen patients received primary radical excision instead of amputation or disarticulation. Among these, 11 patients had a local recurrence and had to undergo amputation secondarily, however, they all died finally. The remaining 4 patients survived for more than 5 years. Among the 6 patients who had lobectomy for pulmonary metastasis, 3 patients survived free of disease for 11, 10, and 10 years, respectively.

DISCUSSION

Surgical ablation shortly after the initial detection of the primary tumor gave disappointing results. Therefore, many efforts have been expended in searching for other methods of treatment for osteosarcoma.

Radiotherapy was the first adjunctive therapy which had a widespread trial. It was learned that there was no favorable change in the result of treatment even by amputation carried out immediately after irradiation, compared to amputation at 6 months later, provided pulmonary metastases were not detected at that time. The only advantage of the delayed amputation was to reduce the number of patients who underwent it, and on that account a high survival rate was seen among those amputees (6).

In recent years radiotherapy has been reviewed from the standpoint of immunology as pulmonary metastatic nodules occasionally showed a slow growth for a short time after radiotherapy of the primary lesion. It was assumed that the necrotic tissue of osteosarcoma probably produced immunogenic substances which increased the host immune response after radiation and displayed an antitumor effect. Based upon this hypothesis radiotherapy with high doses of 10,000 to 20,000 rad was tried by Itami et al. (4). He demonstrated an improvement in the survival rate without radical surgery after radiotherapy.

The absence of an intima in the sinusoids and capillary network of osteosarcoma has been demonstrated by Lagergren (9) and may be related to the high incidence of spontaneous bleeding and necrosis within the tumor as well as to its early hematogenous dissemination. The growth potential of tumor emboli in the lung tends to parallel the activity of the primary tumor. Therefore, treatment should be aimed at the inhibition of the primary tumor and the tumor emboli.

Since the systemic administration of older anticancer agents was thought to be an ineffective method, it was desirable to minimize the systemic toxicity and to expose the primary tumor cell to higher concentrations of these agents. Hence isolation perfusion therapy (14), utilizing a circuit, was started in 1960 in the Department of Orthopaedic Surgery of the University of Tokyo as a preoperative procedure combined with radical operation which took place 2 weeks after the perfusion.

In 1973, Tateishi et al. (13) investigated the results of perfusion in 75 patients with osteosarcoma. According to their report, the 5-year survivors numbered 16 of 50 cases which were followed for more than 5 years and the expected 5-year survival rate of that series by applying the life table technique was 31.2%. They suspected that the reason for the considerable improvement of the survival rate might be due to some kind of humoral or cell-mediated immunological reaction that developed during the 2 weeks after perfusion.

Okai (11) demonstrated experimentally with rats that the delayed amputation or non-amputation group showed a high survival rate compared with the early amputation group. It seems that Tateishi has recently modified the proposed method by supplementing with continuous regional intra-arterial infusion therapy between perfusion and amputation.

Since 1950, when Klopp (7) first reported on intra-arterial infusion in the treatment of malignant tumor, many authors have discussed this technique, emphasizing its remarkable local effects and minimal systemic side-effects. Sullivan and Zurek (12) reported success by using long-term, continuous, intra-arterial infusions in patients with malignancies of the tongue, maxilla, and skin. In addition, Herter et al. (5) have recorded similar results using intermittent, high dose, intra-arterial injections for these tumors. These reports suggested that the treatment of malignant bone tumors might also be improved by the intra-arterial infusion of antimetabolic agents. In 1963, Akahoshi (2) first carried out this infusion chemotherapy combined with surgery for the treatment of malignant tumors of the limbs in Japan. High concentrations of anticancer agents can be infused and the infusion period was more than 3 weeks in duration, the estimated 5-year survival rate being 42.8%.

In this report, 53 cases treated relatively recently in 3 hospitals were investigated. The relative 5-year survival rate was 42.9%. Three of 6 patients who had pulmonary metastasis and underwent pulmonary surgery were alive and free of disease by the

5-year follow-up date. This contributed to the 5-year survival rate. In the treatment of pulmonary metastasis, aggressive pulmonary resection should be performed, if possible, unless there are signs of inoperability. Fifteen cases in this series underwent initial wide resection of the lesion and 11 of these died within a few years. If they had been treated with initial amputation, some of them would have lived longer and the 5-year survival rate would have improved to more than 42.9%.

These results are very encouraging although the number of patients treated was too small for any final evaluation.

REFERENCES

1. Akahoshi, Y., Takeuchi, S., Chen, S. H., Nishimoto, T., Kikuike, A., Yonezawa, H., and Yamamuro, T. The results of surgical treatment combined with intra-arterial infusion of anti-cancer agents in osteosarcoma. *Clin. Orthop.*, **120**, 103–109 (1976).

2. Akahoshi, Y. Intra-arterial infusion combined with surgery for the treatment of malignant bone tumor. *Rynsho Seikei Geka (Clin. Orthop. Surg. Japan)*, **2**, 539–549 (1967) (in Japanese).

3. Aoike, I. Analysis of the long-term survival in osteosarcoma. *Rynsho Seikei Geka (Clin. Orthop. Surg. Japan)*, **2**, 565–569 (1967) (in Japanese).

4. Aoki, H., Itami, Y., Akamatsu, N., Matsuura, Y., Fukushima, M., and Mochizuki, S. Cell-mediated tumor immunity after high dose radiotherapy for a long period of time in osteosarcoma. *Nippon Seikei Geka Gakkaishi (J. Japan. Orthop. Assoc.)*, **50**, 767–768 (1976) (in Japanese).

5. Herter, F. P., Markowitz, A. M., and Feind, C. R. Cancer chemotherapy by continuous intra-arterial infusion of anti-metabolites. *Am. J. Surg.*, **105**, 628–639 (1963).

6. Herman, D. S. Radiotherapy in osteosarcoma. *Clin. Orthop.*, **111**, 71–75 (1975).

7. Klopp, C. T., Alford, T. C., Bateman, J., Berry, G. N., and Winship, T. Fractionated intra-arterial cancer chemotherapy with methyl bis amine hydrochloride; a preliminary report. *Ann. Surg.*, **132**, 811–832 (1950).

8. Kurihara, N. Computing method of the relative survival rate. *Gan-no-Rinsho (Cancer Clinic)*, **11**, 628–632 (1965).

9. Langren, C., Lindbom, A., and Soderberg, G. The blood vessel of osteogenic sarcoma, histologic, angiographic, and microradiographic studies. *Acta Radiol.*, **55**, 161–176 (1961).

10. Lucias, F. S. and Eugene, R. M. Chemotherapy of osteosarcoma. *Clin. Orthop.*, **111**, 101–104 (1975).

11. Okai, K. Experimental tumor therapy by regional perfusion. *J. Bone Joint Surg.*, **49-A**, 1329–1344 (1967).

12. Sullivan, R. D. and Zurek, W. Z. Chemotherapy for liver cancer by protracted ambulatory infusion. *J. Am. Med. Assoc.*, **194**, 481–486 (1965).

13. Tateishi, A., Sekine, K., Ohno, T., and Abe, M. Perfusion chemotherapy of osteosarcoma —a clinical study on 75 cases. *Minerva Oncol.*, (1976) in press.

14. Tateishi, A. The results of regional perfusion in the treatment of osteosarcoma. *Nippon Gan Chiryo Gakkaishi (J. Japan. Cancer Ther.)*, **6**, 632–638 (1971) (in Japanese).

15. The incidence of bone tumor in Japan. Annual report in 1974, National Cancer Center.

CHEMOTHERAPY OF LEUKEMIA AND LYMPHOMA WITH SPECIAL REFERENCE TO REMISSION INDUCTION THERAPY AND SURVIVALS

Kiyoji Kimura,[1],[2] Yasunobu Sakai,[1],[3] Chihiro Konda,[1]
Teruo Sakano,[1] Masanori Shimoyama,[1] and
Takeshi Kitahara[1]

Department of Internal Medicine, National Cancer Center Hospital[1]

Chemotherapy of leukemia and lymphoma has progressed with the discovery of new anticancer agents. In particular, application of vinca alkaloids and daunomycin for acute leukemia, vinca alkaloids, bleomycin, and adriamycin for malignant lymphoma, and combinations of them enables us to discuss the effects of chemotherapy from the viewpoints of remission rate and survivals in leukemia and lymphoma. Childhood leukemia and Hodgkin's disease are now most sensitive to chemotherapeutic agents and are expected to be a curable disease in the near future. However, acute myelogenous leukemia and non-Hodgkin's lymphoma are moderately sensitive to chemotherapeutic agents alone. For these reasons, VEMP (vincristine, endoxan, 6-mercaptopurine (6MP), prednisolone) and DCMP (daunomycin, cytosine arabinoside, 6MP, prednisolone) combination chemotherapy for acute myelogenous leukemia have been tried and established. Particularly, DCMP therapy for acute myelogenous leukemia in adults showed a more than 60% complete remission rate and prolongation of survival. In the treatment of non-Hodgkin's lymphoma, VEMP and BEMP (bleomycin, endoxan, 6MP, prednisolone) combination therapy are most effective; by alternative use of VEMP and BEMP a complete remission rate of 80% was observed. However, the pleomorphic type of reticulum cell sarcoma and T-cell lymphoma showed resistance to chemotherapy. In order to control this type of lymphoma, VEP-AB (adriamycin and bleomycin) combination therapy has been planned by the leukemia and lymphoma cooperative studies group of National Hospitals in Japan.

Chemotherapy of leukemia and lymphoma has progressed with the discovery of new anticancer agents. Furthermore, the widespread application of combination chemotherapy enables us to discuss the effects of chemotherapy from the viewpoint of remission rate and survivals in leukemia and lymphoma patients. The remission rate, remission duration, and survival in childhood leukemia have been remarkably im-

---

[1] Tsukiji 5-1-1, Chuo-ku, Tokyo 104, Japan (木村禧代二, 坂井保信, 近田千尋, 坂野輝夫, 下山正徳, 北原武志).

[2] Present address: National Nagoya Hospital, Sannomaru 4-1, Kita-ku, Nagoya 460, Japan.

[3] Present address: Tokyo Metropolitan Komagome Hospital, Komagome 3-18-22, Bunkyo-ku, Tokyo 113, Japan.

proved and it could become a curable disease in the near future. In adult leukemia and malignant lymphoma, particularly acute myelogenous leukemia (AML) and non-Hodgkin's lymphoma, most investigators have been trying remission induction, consolidation, and maintenance therapy to get higher remission rates and longer remission durations. Generally speaking, the efficacy of these will be predicted in two ways. One is related to empirically clinical experience refering to previous studies, the other is based on *in vitro* and *in vivo* experimental results using tissue culture techniques and animal experiments. In this paper, the clinical results of multicombination therapy in the treatment of leukemia and lymphoma in Japan will be discussed.

Chemotherapy of Leukemia

1. Acute leukemia in adults

The progress of chemotherapy in acute leukemia depends on the development of efficient new agents on the one hand and a combination of existing antileukemic agents on the other hand to improve the remission rate. In other words, not only new agents, but also an efficient combination chemotherapy are the most important things in the treatment of acute leukemia. In Japan, combination chemotherapy of acute leukemia started in 1955 with a protocol of 6-mercaptopurine (6MP) and prednisolone (*8*). The basic idea depends on the accumulated knowledge from the chemotherapy of pulmonary tuberculosis. The results were reported by Hibino and Kimura in the 8th International Congress of Hematology in Tokyo, 1960 (*8, 13*). Since then, by development of new anti-leukemic agents such as endoxan (cyclophosphamide), vinca alkaloids, cytosine arabinoside, cyclocytidine, daunomycin, and adriamycin, various kinds of combination chemotherapy such as EMP (combination of endoxan, 6MP, and prednisolone), CMP (cytosine arabinoside, 6MP, prednisolone), DCP (daunomycin, cytosine arabinoside, prednisolone), VEMP (vincristine, endoxan, 6MP, prednisolone), DCMP (daunomycin, cytosine arabinoside, 6MP, prednisolone), ACMP (adriamycin, cytosine arabinoside, 6MP, prednisolone), and NCMP (neocarzinostatin, cytosine arabinoside, 6MP, prednisolone) have been applied to acute leukemia (*14, 18, 20*). From the international viewpoint of chemotherapy of acute leukemia, VAMP (vincristine, methotrexate, 6MP, prednisone) started in 1963 (*6*). At the present time, many combination therapies including vinca alkaloids, daunomycin, adriamycin, cytosine arabinoside and so on have been applied to acute leukemia all over the world. In this paper, the effect of VEMP and DCMP that originated in Japan will be reported.

1) VEMP therapy

Remission rate: VEMP therapy (vincrisitine 0.04 mg/kg/week, i.v., endoxan 2 mg/kg/day, i.v., 6MP 2 mg/kg/day, p.o., prednisolone 0.6–0.8 mg/kg/day, p.o.) was deviced in the National Cancer Center Hospital in 1968. Remission rates in remission induction therapy for adult AML patients according to the course of therapy are shown in Table I. The complete remission rate was 48.0% which is higher than that of other combinations. If the partial remission rate is included, the remission rate is as high as 61.5%. Complete and partial remission rates according to the number of courses of therapy is 33.3% and 16.6%, in the initial course of therapy, respectively, 55.5% and 11.1% in the second course after the first relapse, and 64.2% and 7.1% in the third

TABLE I. Response Rate to Chemotherapy in Adults with Acute Myelocytic Leukemia

Schedule	No. of courses	Course of treatment					Remission rate
		1	2	3	4	5	
Prednisolone	6	3(2)[a]/4	0/1	0/1	—	—	50.0 (33.3)[b]
(large dose)	4	2(2)/2	0/1	—	—	0/1	50.0 (50.0)
MP	16	3(3)/6	1/7	—	1(1)/2	0/1	31.3 (25.0)
EMP	16	4(2)/10	1(1)/3	0/1	1/1	1(1)/1	43.8 (25.0)
VEMP	52	6(4)/12	12(10)/18	10(9)/14	3(2)/5	1(1)/1	61.5 (48.0)
VAMP	11	1/4	1/4	1(1)/2	—	0/1	27.3 (9.0)
DCMP	12	2(2)/2	0/2	0/3	0/1	1(1)/4	25.5 (25.0)
DAMP	6	1(1)/2	0/1	—	0/1	0/2	16.7 (16.7)
Other single drug	21	4(1)/8	0/1	2/3	2/4	0/5	38.1 (4.8)
Other combination	60	3(2)/7	5(2)/17	0/9	1(1)/8	5(3)/19	23.3 (15.0)
Total	204	29(19)/57	20(14)/55	13(10)/33	8(6)/22	8(6)/37	38.2 (25.9)

( )[a], complete remission case ; ( )[b], complete remission rate.

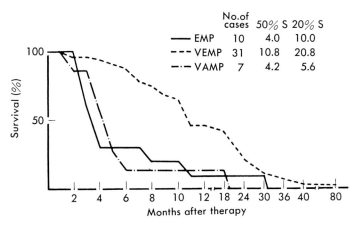

FIG. 1. Effect of main therapy on survival in adults with AML

therapy course after a second relapse. It is considered that these remission rates have nothing to do with the number of courses of therapy.

Remission duration: Fifty percent duration periods of remission of cases of complete remission is 120 days for MP, 135 days for EMP, and 56 days for VEMP in the first induction therapy. The remission duration of cases with complete remission for VEMP, showed no significant differences between the initial and post-first relapse group. This VEMP therapy was evaluated by the envelope method in the 5th Cooperative Study Group of the National Hospital in Japan.

Survival: Survivals in adult AML according to the main therapy are shown in Fig. 1. Fifty percent survival is 4.0 months for EMP and 4.2 months for VAMP, whereas it remarkably increases to 10.8 months in the cases with VEMP. This prolongation of survival for VEMP also shows over 2-fold increase in 20% of survivals in comparison with EMP and VAMP. There is hardly any need to refer to the significance of remission, particularly complete remission, which influences survival in acute leukemia. Survival

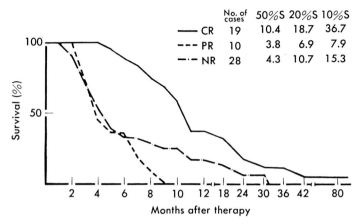

Fig. 2. Effect of response to initial therapy on survival in adults with AML
CR, complete remission; PR, partial remission; NR, no response.

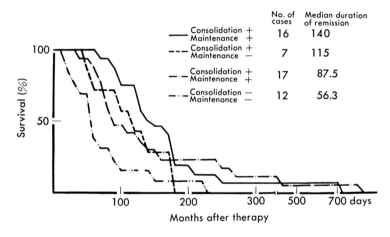

Fig. 3. Comparative effect of consolidation and maintenance therapy on remission duration in adults with AML

according to degree of remission is shown in Fig. 2. Fifty percent survival for cases of complete remission was 10.4 months, whereas it markedly decreased to 3.8 months and 4.3 months, respectively, in cases of partial remission and no response. To prolong the remission duration, many kinds of consolidation and maintenance therapies are conducted. Concerning the duration of remission according to related consolidation, the median duration of remission was 140 days for the cases with both consolidation and maintenance therapy; however, it decreased to 56.3 days for the cases without both consolidation and maintenance therapy, as shown in Fig. 3.

2) *DCMP therapy*

From the basis of experimental results by Hoshino (*10*), the DCMP protocol A was started by Ogawa *et al.* in 1969. The initial protocol consisted of daily administration of prednisolone, 30 mg, p.o.; 6MP, 50–100 mg, p.o.; cytosine arabinoside, 40 mg, i.v.; and daunomycin, 20 mg, i.v. every other day until achieving complete remission.

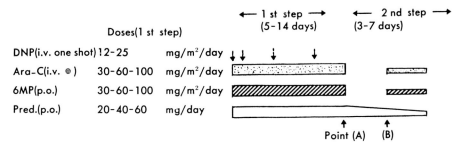

FIG. 4.   DCMP two-step protocol for acute non-lymphatic leukemia (ANLL)
◎ i.v. drip infusion, 2–4 hr/day; Ara-C, cytosine arabinoside; Pred, prednisolone.

While performing this protocol it was occasionally difficult to continue the regimen, mainly due to hemorrhage and infection caused by accompanying severe aplastic bone marrow. Therefore, the protocol was revised regarding the differences of the cell cycle between normal hematopoietic cells and leukemic cells, particularly drawing attention to the lesser damage and faster recovery of remaining normal hematopoietic cells in the bone marrow. This protocol was modified by Ogawa himself (20), Uzuka (23), and Yamada (24) and finally by the leukemia cooperation study group supported by a Grant-in-Aid for Cancer Research from the Ministry of Health and Welfare. The protocol of this group is shown in Fig. 4.

Remission rate: The complete remission rate reported by Uzuka, Ogawa, and Yamada was 83.9%, 60%, and 63% in adult AML, respectively. These have been some of the highest complete remission rates in the world in the treatment of adult AML.

Duration of complete remission: Fifty percent duration periods of complete remission by Uzuka was 46 weeks of DCMP treatment. The longest duration of remission was 177 weeks and this patient maintained complete remission for 21 weeks after the discontinuation of therapy. After DCMP therapy, recurrence mostly appeared within 2 years, in other words, after 2 years' remission, the risk of recurrence will decrease. That reported by Ogawa is 26 weeks.

Survivals: Survival after therapy of all cases with DCMP by Uzuka ranged between 3 weeks and 177 weeks. Fifty percents survival was 53 weeks as shown in Fig. 5. There

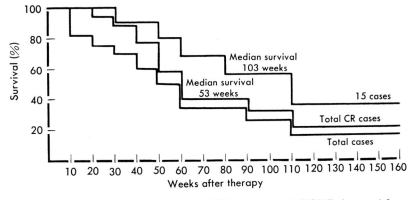

FIG. 5.   Duration of survival in adult ANLL treated with DCMP therapy (after Dr. Uzuka)

is no difference between survivals of total and total complete remission cases with DCMP, because of high complete remission rate. However, survival in the latest 15 cases with DCMP 2-step protocol is 103 weeks. From these results, prolongation of life span in adult AML might be expected in near future. In the DCMP protocol started as a cooperative leukemia study group in 1977, complete remission was observed in 45 of 81 cases of AML in adults. The complete remission rate was 55.5%. This protocol is widely used in the treatment of AML in adults in Japan.

2. *Acute leukemia in children*

The chemotherapy of acute leukemia in children shows great progress in Japan (*7, 11*). In this paper, the treatment schedule and survival rate in the Tokyo Childhood Leukemia Study Group are shown in Figs. 6 and 7. Childhood leukemia might be considered as curable disease from these survivals.

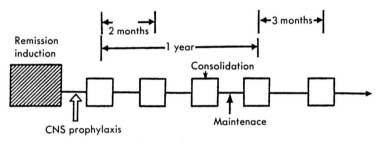

FIG. 6.   Treatment schedules for childhood leukemia (after Dr. Ise)
  i.th., intrathecal; VCR, vincristine; MTX, methotrexate; CNS, central nervous system.

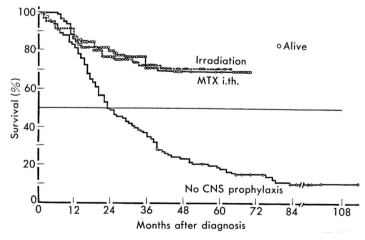

FIG. 7.   Survival rate of acute lymphatic leukemia in children (after Dr. Ise)

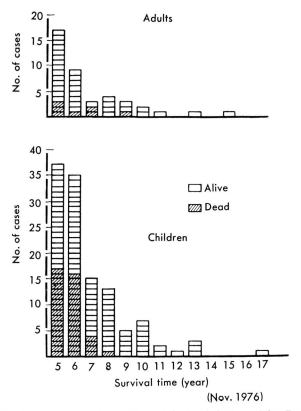

FIG. 8.   Long-term survivors with acute leukemia in Japan (after Dr. Yamada)

3.   Five-year survivors with acute leukemia in Japan

It has been admitted that the present-day treatment of acute leukemia is capable not only of producing remission and thus leading to a prolonged period of normal health, but also actually to extend the total survival time. In the meantime, we have rarely seen patients who survived an extraordinarily long time. It will be of interest to study whether the long-term survivors of acute leukemia might provide appreciable differences in host-tumor-drug relationship as compared to those of ordinary cases. In May 1964, Yamada (25) initiated studies on long-term survivors with acute leukemia by sending an inquiry form to hospitals that have more than 200 beds in Japan. At that time, 3 patients with a 5-year survival were reported. In August 1971, they made a second survey and, at that time, 50 patients with a 5-year survival were collected. They then visited each hospital that had sent them a report of 5-year survivors and checked their records and the blood specimen. Furthermore, in 1976 they made a third survey and 178 cases of 5-year survivors were collected and analyzed from the viewpoint of tumor-drug-host relationship (25). Only two points will be introduced in this paper concerning the alive and dead cases confirmed by follow-up study.

1)   Age and type of the disease

As shown in Fig. 8, out of 178 patients with a 5-year survival, 137 cases are children under the age of 14 and 41 cases are adults. Thirty-eight of 50 patients in the

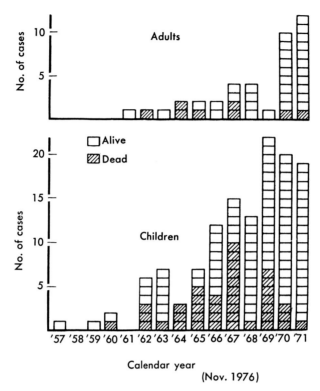

Fɪɢ. 9. Chronological changes in number of long-term survivors (after Dr. Yamada)

survey in 1971, *i.e.*, 76% of cases, were those under the age of 10, and the rest of the cases were distributed sporadically in the older age groups. In contrast, in the survey in 1976, 102 of 178 cases, *i.e.*, 57.6% of cases, were those under the age of 10. The number of patients with adult leukemia are increasing in Japan, as shown in this figure.

2) *Chronological changes in number of long-term survivors*

As shown in Fig. 9, 5-year survivors have shown a yearly increase in number, particularly in 1962 in children and 1970 in adults. Between 1962 and 1965, 7 to 9 patients were reported each year, and in 1966, it increased to 14 cases, while in 1971 it increased to 31 cases. Such an increase in 5-year survivors is attributed to the discovery of new antileukemic agents and the device of new combination therapy, as well as consolidation and maintenance therapy.

4. *Summary and discussion*

In Japan, Hibino and Kimura reported that 50% survival of patients with acute leukemia is less than 2 months and all patients died at less than 6 months in 1951. However, starting with methotrexate in 1948, 6MP (1953), cyclophosphamide (1960), and vincristine (1962), cytosine arabinoside (1963), and daunomycin (1965), it became possible to discuss the remission rate, remission duration, and prolongation of survival. However, even when temporary remission was obtained with such drugs, 2-year survivors were less than 20% in adult leukemia. Concerning 5-year survivors, it is not difficult to assume that there is a certain difference between common leukemic cases and various factors of the host-tumor-drug relationship of the long-term survivors. Burchenal reported 71 acute leukemia cases that survived for more than 5 years after establishment of diagnosis, and that most of them were those of lymphatic leukemia, with children numbering 53 (74.6%) (3). Similarly, in Yamada's series in 1971, 40 of 50 patients with a 5-year survival were children under the age of 14 and two-thirds of patients have the lymphoblastic type. In general, 82% of cases had peroxidase-negative leukemic cells. These data make it clear that the age factor as well as type of disease play a great role in producing long term survivors. In reviewing the therapy used, it can be seen that almost all were given adrenal steroids, 6MP, or methotrexate or combination therapy. The first reported 5-year survival rate was that by Zuelzer (1968) (26), who treated 229 consecutive children with acute lymphoblastic leukemia; 4.3% of these children were alive at 5 years. In the 227 patients seen by members of the acute leukemia group B in 1960 and 1961 (1), approximately 2% survived 5 years; for patients treated in 1962 and 1963, the 5-year survival rate was 5%; and for those treated in 1964 and 1965, it was 10%. Bernard (2) has reported that 12 of 52 patients given intensive combination therapy during 1964 and 1965 have survived over 4.5 years. There have been no reports on a nation-wide scale based on the underlying leukemic population in a given country. Yamada's data indicated that it was 0.13% in childhood cases in 1958 and it increased to 1.55%, whereas in adult cases, there has been no significant increase, being 0.097% in 1966. Nevertheless, the increasing rate of survival at 3 years in the more recently treated series of patients continues; therefore, one might expect at least as high a percentage of 5-year survivors in these group. Burchenal (4) cited that it would seem reasonable to suggest that in the patient with acute leukemia who survived over 7 years from the diagnosis of his disease and had had no evidence of leukemia for the previous 4 years, it should be reasonably safe to discontinue treatment on the assumption that all leukemic cells had been eradicated. In the Japanese series of 5-year survivors, 19 patients who have survived for more than 10 years are all living, well, and with no evidence of disease and these patients have had no episodes of relapse. On the other hand, only 2 patients died among 24 patients who continued in initial remission for more than 5 years. It should be emphasized also that there has been only one relapsed case out of 14 patients who had continuous maintenance therapy over 5 years, whereas the majority of cases with death or relapse were fonud in a group of patients who had maintenance therapy for less than 5 years. From these data, it can be stated that it will be safe to discontinue treatment when the patient with acute leukemia has survived over 5 years on continuous maintenance therapy with no evidence of leukemia, and also when the patient has survived over 8 years from the diagnosis of his disease with no evidence of disease regardless of the therapy hitherto used. In conclusion, the complete remission rate is increasing and the remission duration is becoming longer. This makes the number of long-term survivors increase in Japan. Furthermore, We would like to emphasize that it is very important to get complete remission such that there are less than 1% of myeloblasts in the bone marrow for increasing the number of long-term survivors in the first induction therapy.

TABLE II. Parameters for Early Diagnosis of Blast Crisis in CML (after Dr. Kitajima)

1. Major parameters
    1) Enlargement of splenomegaly
    2) Myeloblasts more than 5% in peripheral blood or bone marrow
    3) Promyelocytes more than 20% in peripheral blood or bone marrow
    4) Multiple Ph[1], other chromosome abnormality
2. Minor parameters
    1) Fever ($>38°$) of unknown cause
    2) Neuralgia of extremities
    3) Hemorrhagic diathesis
    4) Anemia ($<300\times10^4$) of unknown cause
    5) Thrombocytopenia ($<10\times10^4$) or thrombocytosis ($>300\times10^4$)
    6) Basophilic leucocytosis more than 20%
    7) Dry tap in bone marrow
    8) CRP positive
    9) Increase of NAP score more than 80%
    10) Swelling of lymph node

Chemotherapy of Chronic Myelogenous Leukemia

The prognosis of chronic myelogenous leukemia (CML) depends strongly upon "blast crisis." More than 150 cases of CML have been treated with chemotherapy by us in the past 30 years' period and 80 cases were terminated by "blast crisis." As a clinician, one of the problems in the treatment of CML is how to prevent "blast crisis" and keep the patient in a chronic stage, another is how to determine the early stage of "blast crisis" and give the effective chemotherapy at the appropriate time, keeping the patient in long remission status. The main agents in Japan for CML are busulfan, mitomycin C, and 6MP. The important point in this treatment is the small amount of busulfan and mitomycin C administered. The mode of action of these two agents belong to the alkylating group, that is, mutagenic agents with which one expects to have a sudden blast crisis. Therefore, administration of high doses must be expected to cause a sudden decrease of WBC and to be followed by rapid recovery from leukopenia, which might trigger "blast crisis". Accordingly, small amounts of busulfan and mitomycin C were administered in order to decrease the WBC slowly and completely reduce splenomegaly with the WBC count slightly higher than normal level, about 15,000/mm³ over a long period. Fifty percent survival of CML patients created in this way, revealed 4.0 years by mitomycin C and 3.3 years by busulfan, there being no difference between these two agents as far as 50% survival is concerned (9). As a prevention of "blast crisis", 6MP alone or in combination with busulfan or mitomycin C was tried, but as yet no difference in the survival curves has occurred. Using a small amount of busulfan for CML, Kinugasa obtained a 50% survival of 5 years (17). This is the most excellent result in Japan. Diagnosis studies on "blast crisis" have been carried out by Kitajima (19); the criteria for "blast crisis" as shown in Table II from the physical and hematological point of view were prepared by him, and blast crisis can be diagnosed by 3 major, or a combination of 2 major and 3 minor parameters. This is the starting point of chemotherapy. The real importance is how to treat the patients with blast crisis. When a VEMP or DCMP combination were applied to case with blast crisis, a remission rate of 30–40% was obtained. The above results strongly indicated the importance of chemotherapy against blast crisis. It is expected that blast crisis will not be the terminal stage of CML in the near future.

Chemotherapy of Malignant Lymphomas

Before reporting the results of chemotherapy of malignant lymphoma, the mortality and pathologically characteristic patterns of malignant lymphoma in Japan will be reported.

1. Mortality of malignant lymphoma

It has been reported that the incidence of malignant lymphoma as well as leukemia is increasing each year all over the world. In Japan, the mortality rate per 100,000 population from non-Hodgkin's lymphoma (reticulum cell sarcoma and lymphosarcoma) was 0.52 in 1950, 1.0 in 1960, 1.43 in 1967, 1.14 in 1973, and 1.17 in 1976. In other words, the mortality rate in 1967 was more than double that of 1950, and from 1967 it has maintained an almost constant level. In more detailed observation of these results, the mortality rate from reticulum cell sarcoma was 0.46 in 1959, 0.82 in 1967, 0.77 in 1973, and 0.77 in 1976. In contrast, that from lymphosarcoma was 0.41 in 1959, 0.43 in 1967, 0.37 in 1973, and 0.39 in 1976. From these results, the increase in the mortality of non-Hodgkin's lymphoma may be attributed to that of reticulum cell sarcoma; this is in contrast to the tendency in other countries. In addition, the mortality from Hodgkin's lymphoma during the period of 1950 to 1976 ranged from 0.40 to 0.58 per 100,000 population showing almost no increase during this 27-year period. However, the incidence of Hodgkin's disease in those over 40 years of age is actually increasing. This mortality rate from malignant lymphoma is different from the tendency in other countries where the mortality from Hodgkin's lymphoma is higher than that in Japan.

2. Histological type of malignant lymphoma

Nineteen hundred forty-one and 1709 cases with malignant lymphoma were collected in Japan in 1963 and 1976, respectively. In 1963, the percentage of reticulum cell sarcoma, lymphosarcoma, and Hodgkin's lymphoma was 60.0, 16.0 and 24.0, and in 1975, was 62.0, 16.7 and 21.4, respectively. It is characteristic that the incidence of non-Hodgkin's lymphoma is very high in Japan. Histological classification of 212 cases with malignant lymphoma in the National Cancer Center Hospital showed 83.1% of cases of non-Hodgkin's lymphoma. Classification of non-Hodgkin's lymphoma by Rappaport's classification showed that 77.3% of the cases consisted of the diffuse type of non-Hodgkin's lymphoma and 22.7% of nodular type.

3. Chemotherapy of malignant lymphoma

The application of vinca alkaloids, bleomycin, and adriamycin to malignant lymphoma enables us to discuss the effects of chemotherapy from the viewpoint of remission rate and survival time. Now, many combination chemotherapies have been reported (5, 12, 15, 22). Our chemotherapy schedule for malignant lymphoma is shown in Fig. 10. VEMP therapy such as the combination of vincristine, endoxan, 6MP, and prednisolone, and BEMP such as a combination of bleomycin, endoxan, 6MP, and

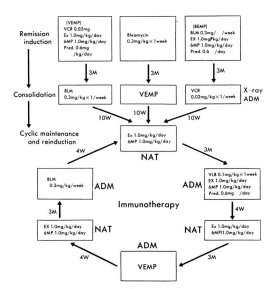

Fig. 10. Chemotherapeutic schedule for malignant lymphoma in adults
EX, endoxan; BLM, bleomycin; NAT, natulan; ADM, adriamycin.

prednisolone are the most common combination chemotherapies for the last 10 years in Japan. The patients who are successufully induced to complete remission by VEMP chemotherapy, further have been treated by another combination therapy including bleomycin as a consolidation therapy. The cases who are successfully induced to complete remission by BEMP combination therapy, further have been treated by combination therapy including vinca alkaloid as a consolidation. Afterwards, the patient has been treated by cyclic maintenance and reconsolidation therapy over a long-term period as shown in this figure. The number of cases and treatment with chemotherapy in the National Cancer Center Hospital are shown in Table III. Remission rates according to the first course of chemotherapy are shown in Table IV. The complete remission rate by VEMP in reticulum cell sarcoma, lymphosarcoma, and Hodgkin's disease are 56%, 56%, and 42%, respectively. Complete remission rates by combination therapy including bleomycin, such as BEMP, in reticulum cell sarcoma is 45%, but in lymphosarcoma with bleomycin, complete remissions were observed in 3 of 4 cases and in Hodgkin's disease, it was observed in 2 of 4 cases. According to our experience including a second course of therapy, bleomycin for Hodgkin's disease might be more effective than vincristine. Furthermore, bleomycin shows cytocidal and concentration-dependent action; also it is time-dependent in a constant concentration according to

TABLE III. Number of Cases and Treatment with Chemotherapy

	RCSA	LSA	HD	Total
No. of cases	182	56	61	299
No. of treatmens	471	164	216	851

RCSA, reticulum cell sarcoma ; LSA, lymphosarcoma ; HD, Hodgkin's disease.

TABLE IV. Remission Rate in First Course Therapy

	RCSA	LSA	HD	Total
VCR	3/4 (3/4)	2/2 (1/2)	9/9 (5/9)	82% (53%) 17
VEMP	77% (56%)	69% (56%)	83% (42%)	76% (54%)
No. of cases	64	16	12	92
VCR (other C.)	63% (50%)	60% (30%)	91% (64%)	69% (49%)
	24	10	11	45
VLB	— (—)	1/1 (0/1)	1/2* (1/2)	2/3 (1/3) 3
VLB combination	1/2 (1/2)	0/1 (0/1)	— (—)	1/3 (1/3) 3
BLM	4/8 (3/8)	2/2 (0/2)	1/2 (1/2)	58% (33%) 12
Oil BLM	1/1 (1/1)	1/1 (1/1)	2/3 (1/3)	4/5 (3/5) 5
BLM combination	73% (45%) 11	3/4 (3/4)	3/4 (2/4)	74% (53%) 19
ADM	— (—)	— (—)	— (—)	— (—)
ADM combination	— (—)	— (—)	— (—)	— (—)
VEPA (B)	1/1 (0/1)	— (—)	— (—)	1/1 (0/1) 1
Others single drug	46% (8%)	4/8 (0/8)	0/2 (0/2)	43% (4%) 23
Other combination	7% (14%) 14	2/4 (1/4)	1/5 (0/5)	17% (13%) 23

( ), complete remission ; V or VCR, vincristine ; E, endoxan ; M, 6 MP ; P, prednisolone ; VLB, vinblastine ; B or BLM, bleomycin ; A or ADM, adriamycin.

TABLE V. Response to VEMP Therapy According to Number of Courses
in Non-Hodgkin's Lymphoma

No. of course	1	2	3	4	5–
Nodular					
Lymphocytic	1/2	0/2	—	—	—
Mixed	1/2	1/1	—	—	—
Histiocytic	1/4	3/6	2/4	—	0/5
Diffuse					
Lymphocytic	3/5	2/11	0/2	0/1	0/2
Mixed	4/5	4/6	—	0/1	0/2
Histiocytic	9/16	5/12	1/6	1/3	1/3
Pleomorphic	6/12	1/4	2/4	0/1	—
Total	25/46 (54%)	16/42 (38%)	5/16 (31%)	1/6 (17%)	1/12 (8%)

CR/total No. of cases.

our experimental results on cell killing kinetics using a soft agar cloning assay. On the basis of these results and others, depo-bleomycin was made and planned for the treatment of malignant lymphoma expecting the time-dependent action of bleomycin. Depo-bleomycin revealed a prolonged high blood concentration compared with that of regular bleomycin. In both Hodgkin's lymphoma and non-Hodgkin's lymphoma with

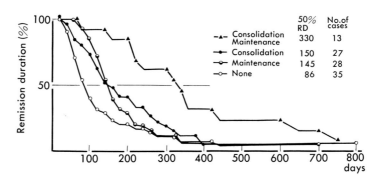

FIG. 11.   Influence of therapy with or without consolidation and/or maintenance
on remission duration in complete remission cases (non-Hodgkin's lymphoma)
RD, remission duration.

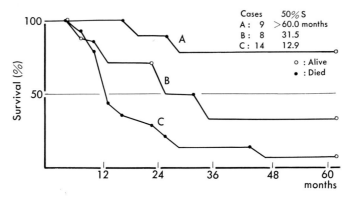

FIG. 12.   Influence of therapy with or without consolidation and/or maintenance
on survival in complete remission cases with Hodgkin's lymphoma (generalized
type)

A, CR cases with consolidation therapy; B, CR cases without consolidation
therapy; C, PR and NR cases. Generalized type, tumor is generalized at first
visit or generalizes in less than 5 months.

depo-bleomycin, the complete remission rate is higher than that in patients with regular
bleomycin regardless of whether the cases had prior chemotherapy (16). In order to
analyze the relationship of response rate to number of courses of chemotherapy, the
complete remission rate by VEMP therapy according to the number of courses of
therapy and histological type in non-Hodgkin's lymphoma were examined. As shown
in Table V, complete remission is observed in 54% in the first course and 17% in the
fourth course of therapy, respectively. The complete remission rate is decreasing with
the number of courses of therapy. In other words, lymphoma cells become resistant
with increasing number of courses of therapy. In order to clarify the effect of consolidation and maintenance therapy, remission duration was analyzed according to cases
with or without consolidation and/or maintenance therapy using complete remission
cases with non-Hodgkin's lymphoma. As shown in Fig. 11, 50% remission duration
of cases with consolidation and maintenance therapy in complete remission cases of

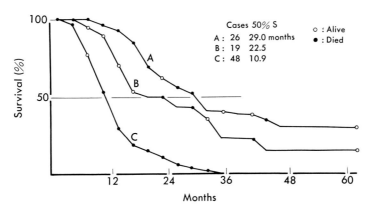

FIG. 13. Influence of therapy with or without consolidation and/or maintenance on survival in complete remission cases with generalized type of reticulum cell sarcoma (A, B, C, see Fig. 12)

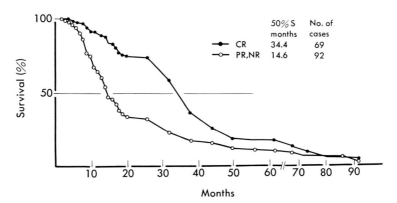

FIG. 14. Survival of complete responders and partial or non-responders (non-Hodgkin's lymphoma)

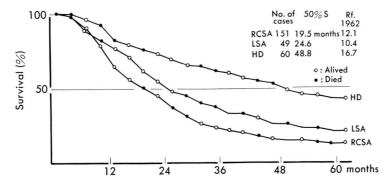

FIG. 15. Survival in reticulum cell sarcoma, lymphosarcoma, and Hodgkin's lymphoma

non-Hodgkin's lymphoma is 330 days; that with consolidation or maintenance therapy is 150 or 145 days, respectively, and that neither consolidation nor maintenance therapy is 86 days. These results show that consolidation and maintenance following induction therapy are very important to obtaining long-term remission periods. Survival time in generalized types (Stage III and IV) of Hodgkin's lymphoma, according to whether the cases had consolidation and/or maintenance therapy, is shown in Fig. 12. In complete remission cases with consolidation, the 50% survival time is over 60 months; in complete remission cases without consolidation, it was 31.5 months, and in partial and non-remission cases, it was 12.9 months. The survival rate with the generalized type of reticulum cell sarcoma according to whether the cases had consolidation and/or maintenance therapy is shown in Fig. 13. In complete remission cases with consolidation, the 50% survival time is 29.0 months, in complete remission cases without consolidation therapy, it is 22.5 months, and in cases without complete remission it was 10.9 months. Survival of complete remission cases and partial or non-remission cases of non-Hodgkin's lymphoma is shown in Fig. 14. The 50% survival times of cases with complete remission is 34.4 months. In cases without complete remission it was 14.6 months. Survival time in all of the cases with reticulum cell sarcoma, lymphosarcoma, and Hodgkin's lymphoma as compared with survival in 1962 is shown in Fig. 15, right upper quadrant. Survival time is prolonged 1.5 or 3 times as compared with that in 1962.

4. Summary and conclusion

The complete remission rate in malignant lymphoma patients following chemotherapy including vinca alkaloids or bleomycin is over 50% or near 50%. Furthermore, according to our results, VEMP shows a 29% complete remission rate in BEMP-resistant cases, and BEMP shows a 12% complete remission rate in VEMP-resistant cases. In other words, at the present time, 60 or 80% of malignant lymphoma has been induced to complete remission by the alternative use of VEMP and BEMP. Other 10% of malignant lymphoma has been treated with adriamycin and L-asparaginase with a 10% complete remission rate. The remaining 10 or 15% of patients have been considered refractory to chemotherapy. The pleomorphic type

TABLE VI. New Protocol for Malignant Lymphoma in National Hospital Group

Schedule		Dose of therapy (days)												
		1	2	3	4	5	6	7	8	9	10	12	13	14
I. VEP-AB														
VCR	0.5–1 mg/m², i.v.	×							×					
EX	200–400 mg/m², i.v.	×							×					
Pred.	30–50 mg/m², i.v.	×	×	×	×	×			×	×	×	×	×	
ADM	20–25 mg/m², i.v.		×											
BLM	10 mg/m², i.v. or i.m.									×				
II. VEPA														
VCR	0.5–1 mg/m²	×							×					
EX	300–400 mg/m², i.v.	×							×					
Pred.	40–50 mg/m², p.o.	×	×	×	×	×			×	×	×	×	×	
ADM	25–30 mg/m²		×							×				

of reticulum cell sarcoma and T-cell lymphoma are examples of this refractory type. For this type of malignant lymphoma, new protocol, VEP-AB and VEPA shown in Table VI is on-going in malignant lymphoma, by a cooperative group of the National Hospital Group in Japan. To get long-term remission(cure), from the viewpoint of the tumor side, drug sensitivity, tumor volume, evolution pattern, and growth rate are very important factors. From the viewpoint of drugs side, more intensive induction and consolidation therapy with the least toxicity and maintenance therapy, and their repetition for a long period, are important. From the host side, early diagnosis and early treatment at an early stage as well as a good immune condition are considered to be important factors.

CONCLUSIONS

In conclusion we would like to emphasize again that to induce a completely complete remission giving a completely disease-free condition from both the tumor and host side in the first course of therapy using the most intensive combination chemotherapy with the least toxicity is very important for the control of blood cancer in the long term and for obtaining cure.

REFERENCES

1. Acute leukemia group B: New treatment schedule with improved survival in childhood leukemia. Intermittent parenteral *vs.* daily oral administration of methotrexate for maintenance of induced remission. *J. Am. Med. Assoc.*, **194**, 75–81 (1965).
2. Bernard, J. Personal communication.
3. Burchenal, J. H. and Murphy, M. L. Long-term survivors in acute leukemia. *Cancer Res.*, **25**, 1491–1494 (1965).
4. Burchenal, J. H. Long-term survivor in acute leukemia. *In* "Proceeding of the International Congress of Leukemia-Lymphoma," ed. by C.J.D. Zerafonetis, Lea & Febiger, Philadelphia, pp. 469–474 (1968).
5. DeVita, V. T., Serpick, A., and Carborne, P. P. Combination chemotherapy in the treatment of advanced Hodgkin's disease. *Ann. Intern. Med.*, **73**, 881, 1 (1970).
6. Freireich, E., Karon, M., and Frei, E. Quadruple combination therapy (VAMP) for acute lymphocytic leukemia in childhood. *Proc. Am. Assoc. Cancer Res.*, **6**, 20 (1965).
7. Fujimoto, M. and Goya, C. Chemotherapy of childhood leukemia-protocol 721, 745 therapy. *Gan-to-Kagakuryoho* (*Cancer Chemother.*), **3**, 399–411 (1976) (in Japanese).
8. Hibino, S. Clinical pathology and chemotherapy of leukemia. *Nippon Ketsueki Gakkaishi* (*Acta Haematol. Japon.*), **18**, 442–462 (1955).
9. Hibino, S. Chemotherapy of leukemia with special reference to mitomycin C and other agents recently originated in Japan. *In* "Proceedings of the VIII International Congress of Hematology," ed. by Organizing Committee, VIIIth International Society of Haematology, Science Council of Japan, Pan-Pacific Press, Tokyo, Vol. 1, pp. 351–359 (1962).
10. Hoshino, A. Combined therapy from point of drug resistance: Resistance of anticancer agents. *In* "The Year Book of Cancer," ed. by Clark et Cumley, Year Book Medical Publishers, Chicago, p. 397 (1970).
11. Ise, T. Personal communication.
12. Kaplan, H. S. On the natural history, treatment and prognosis of Hodgkin's disease. Harvey Lecture, Ser. 64, 1968–1969, Academic Press, New York, pp. 215–259 (1970).

13. Kimura, K. Clinical and hematological patterns influencing the chemotherapeutic effects of acute leukemia. *In* "Proceeding of the VIIIth International Congress of Hematology," ed. by Organizing Committee, VIIIth International Society of Hematology, Science Council of Japan, Pan-Pacific Press, Tokyo, Vol. 1, pp. 488–493 (1962).

14. Kimura, K. Chemotherapy of leukemia. *In* "Proceeding of the 16th General Assembly of the Japan Medical Congress," Tosho-Insatsu Co., Tokyo, Vol. 3, pp. 540–550 (1963) (in Japanese).

15. Kimura, K. Chemotherapy of malignant lymphoma with special reference to the effect of bleomycin and sequential therapy of bleomycin and vinca alkaloids. *In* "Leukämien und maligne Lymphome," ed. by A. Stacher, Urban & Schwaszerberg, München, pp. 418–424 (1973).

16. Kimura, K. Clinical studies with bleomycin in Japan. *In* "Bleomycin Seminar in NCI," pp. 41–58 (1974).

17. Kinugasa, E. Treatment of chronic leukemia. *Ketsueki-to-Myakukan (Blood and Vessel)*, **2**, 259–263 (1971) (in Japanese).

18. Kitajima, K., Kamimura, O., and Hiraki, K. Neocarzinostatin, a new chemotherapeutic approach to acute leukemia. *Nippon Ketsueki Gakkaishi (Acta Haematol. Japon.)*, **37**, 316–328 (1974).

19. Kitajima, K., Ishizaki, M., Nagao, T., Takahashi, I., Kinoshita, H., Shimada, A., Moriwaki, Y., and Uemura, Ch. Clinical studies on early diagnosis and treatment of blast crisis of chronic myelogenous leukemia. *Rinsho Ketsueki (Japan. J. Clin. Hematol.)*, **13**, 560–568 (1972) (in Japanese).

20. Ogawa, M. and Hoshino, A. DCMP therapy in acute leukemia—Experimental and clinical study. *Nippon Ketsueki Gakkaishi (Acta Haematol. Japon.)*, **37**, 108–112 (1974).

21. Sakai, Y. and Sakano, T. Chemotherapy of acute myelocytic leukemia in adults. *Nippon Ketsueki Gakkaishi (Acta Haematol. Japon.)*, **37**, 324–334 (1974).

22. Ultman, J. E. and Nixon, D. D. The therapy of lymphoma, *Seminars Hematol.*, **6**, 376 (1969).

23. Uzuka, Y. and Ryo, M. Remission induction and maintenance-DCMP Protocol. *Gan-to-Kagakuryoho (Cancer Chemother.)*, **2**, 198–208 (1975) (in Japanese).

24. Yamada, K. On multicombination therapy (DCMP) of acute leukemia. *Saishin Igaku (Modern Medicine)*, **28**, 867 (1975) (in Japanese).

25. Yamada, K. and Uetani, T. Five-year survivors with acute leukemia in Japan. *Nippon Ketsueki Gakkaishi (Acta Haematol. Japon.)*, **37**, 335–343 (1974).

26. Zuelzer, W. W. Therapy of acute leukemia in childhood. *In* "Proceedings of the International Congress of Leukemia-Lymphoma," ed. by C. J. D. Zerafonetis, Lea & Febiger, Philadelphia, pp. 451–461 (1968).

GANN Monograph on Cancer Research 22, 1979

CHILDHOOD MALIGNANT TUMORS IN JAPAN

Cancer Study Group for Malignant Tumors in Children[*1]

Masanobu Ishida,[*2] Ikuo Okabe, Ken Morita, Morio Kasai,
Shigenori Sawaguchi, Takashi Ueda, Noboru Kobayashi,
Toru Ise, Yoshiyuki Hanawa, Taro Akabane,
Tadasu Izawa, and Tadashi Sawada,

Department of Surgery, Shōwa University School of Medicine[*2]

The data presented here were prepared and submitted by the group (Ishida) supported by Grant-in-aid from Japanese Ministry of Health and Welfare, 1975.

1. Solid Tumors: During the years between 1963 and 1972, 403 cases of malignant solid tumors (neuroblastoma 239, primary liver cell carcinoma 70, and nephroblastoma 94) were seen by members of the group and their overall 2-year survival rates were 29% in neuroblastoma, 24% in primary liver cell carcinoma, and 50% in nephroblastoma. Those survival rates were analyzed according to the factors which were thought to influence their prognosis.

2. Acute Leukemia: A total of 145 cases of acute leukemia were seen in 4 years, namely 1957, 1962, 1967, and 1972 and their remission rates were 11.5% in 1957, 38.5% 1962, 54.1% 1967, and 88.1% 1972. Also analyzed were the post-treatment complication rate.

This communication contains data quoted from the Annual Report of the Cancer Research, Ministry of Health and Welfare, 1975. The data were prepared and submitted by the group (Ishida) organized especially to improve diagnostic accuracy and prognosis of malignant tumors in infancy and childhood.

Solid Tumors

During the years between 1963 and 1972, 403 cases of malignant solid tumors (neuroblastoma 239, primary liver cell carcinoma 70, and nephroblastoma 94) were seen by group members who were from 13 to 16 institutions in Japan, and 2-year survival rates of those patients were analyzed according to the factors which were thought to influence their prognosis, namely, age, stage of the disease, length of history before treatment, tumor histological types, and different methods of treatment.

Overall 2-year survival rates were 29% in neuroblastoma, 24% in primary liver cell carcinoma, and 50% in nephroblastoma.

In the ensuing discussion, a figure in the parenthesis means 2-year survival rate.

[*1] This group was supported by Grant-in-Aid from the Ministry of Health and Welfare of Japan, 1975.

[*2] Hatanodai 1-5-8, Shinagawa-ku, Tokyo 142, Japan (石田正統, 岡部郁夫, 森田 建, 葛西森夫, 沢口 重徳, 植田 隆, 小林 登, 伊勢 泰, 塙 嘉之, 赤羽太郎, 井沢 道, 沢田 淳).

TABLE I. Age and Prognosis

Age in years	0 Less than 6 months	0 Between 6 and 12 months	1	2	3	4	5	6	7	8	9	10-	Total
Neuroblastoma	26/37 70%	15/29 52%	10/47 21%	5/42 12%	1/20	1/14	1/5	1/8	2/8	0/2	0/1	0/3	61/216
	62%		14%										29%
Nephroblastoma	5/5 100%	6/13 46%	15/22 68%	7/13 54%	4/11 36%	3/7 43%	0/1	0/7	1/1	1/2	1/1	0/3	43/86
	61%		47%										50%
Primary liver cell carcinoma	7/15 46%	5/15 33%	2/9	2/6	0/7	0/1	1/2	0/4	0/2	0/3	0/4	0/2	17/70
	40%		13%										24%

No. of survivors/all cases. 2-Year survival rate in %.

1. Age (Table I)

Neuroblastoma: Prognosis of patients less than one year old (62%) were better than those of over one year old (14%). Especially high were the ones of patients less than 6 months old (70%).

Primary liver cell carcinoma: Two-year survival rate was 40% in patients less than one year old and 13% in patients over one year old.

Nephroblastoma: The highest survival rate (100%) was obtained in patients less than 6 months old and this was followed by patients between one and 2 years old (68%). Two-year survival rate of patients between 6 months and 12 months (46%) was slightly worse, although the reason is unknown. Even up to 4 years old, 36% with a 2-year survival rate was obtained.

2. Stage of the disease (Table II) (1, 5)

In all kinds of tumors in general, there was an inverse relationship between stage of the disease and 2-year survival rate, so that as the disease progressed, the survival rate tended to decline.

Neuroblastoma: In contrast to the above general statement, even advanced disease such as Stage IVs or IVb showed relatively high 2-year survival rates (65% in the former and 30% in the latter). Many of the survivors, however, were less than 6 months old (8 out of 11 with IVs and 5 out of 6 with IVb).

As to the origin of the tumor, adrenal or retropertitoneal tumor showed worse 2-year survival rates (26% altogether) than intrathoracic, pelvic, or cervical tumor (53% altogether).

Primary liver cell carcinoma: Although the reason is unknown, the 2-year survival rate of patients with Stage I disease (33%) was poor, contrary to what might have been expected. However, it was remarkable that there was one survivor even with Stage IV disease.

TABLE II. Stage of the Disease and Prognosis

A. Neuroblastoma

I	14/14	100%
II	10/16	63%
III	18/48	38%
IV A	3/80	4%⎫ 9%
B	6/20	30%⎭
IV s	11/17	65%
Total	62/195	32%

I, Localized to the organ of origin; II, infiltrated through the capsule, but not beyond the midline; III, infiltrated beyond the midline or with contralateral lymph node metastasis; IV, distant meta stasis; IVa, distant metastasis except skin, liver, or bone marrow; IVb, III with skin, liver, or bone marrow metastasis; IVs, I or II with skin, liver, or bone marrow metastasis (1, 5).

B. Nephroblastoma

I	23/26	89%
II	12/20	60%
III	6/19	31%
IV	1/11	9%
V	1/4	25%
Total	43/86	50%

I, Localized to kidney; II, infiltrated to perirenal tissue; III, infiltrated to neighboring organs in the peritoneal cavity; IV, distant metastasis; V, bilateral (1, 5).

C. Primary liver cell carcinoma

I	2/6	33%
II	9/15	60%
III	5/20	25%
IV	1/29	3%
Total	17/70	14%

I, Localized to one segment; II, localized to lobe, right or left; III, involvement of all segments except one; IV, involvement of all segments or to the portal area which preclude resection; other factors such as peritoneal involvement, vascular invasion, lymph node metastasis, and organ metastasis are also taken into account in deciding stages (1, 5).

No. of survivors/all cases. 2-Year survival rate in %.

Nephroblastoma: As in primary liver cell carcinoma, it was also remarkable that one case of Stage V disease survived.

3. Length of history before treatment

Neuroblastoma: No definite relationship between length of history before treatment and 2-year survival rate was found, contrary to what might have been expected. Thus, it seemed that a longer history of symptoms before treatment did not necessarily mean a worse prognosis.

Primary liver cell carcinoma: The same statement as described in neuroblastoma is also applied to this tumor.

Nephroblastoma: In this tumor, the shorter the length of history before treatment, the better the prognosis. Patients with Stage I disease who came to treatment less than one month after the occurrence of symptoms showed a 2-year survival rate of 100%.

4. Tumor histological type (2–4)

Neuroblastoma: There was no difference in survival rate between neuroblastoma (30%) and ganglioneuroblastoma (36%). However, neuroblastoma of a rosette-forming type showed a higher survival rate (43%) than the one of a round cell type (14%). In ganglioneuroblastoma, the well-differentiated type showed a better survival rate (86%) than the mixed type (19%).

Primary liver cell carcinoma: The highest survival rate (42%) was obtained in hepatoblastoma of the well-differentiated type and this was followed by the poorly differentiated type on (13%). No patient with adult type liver cell carcinoma survived.

Nephroblastoma: No definite relationship between histological type and prognosis was seen.

5. *Methods of treatment*

A relationship between the method of treatment and prognosis was studied, while dividing the patients into 2 groups, namely, patients who had surgery only and patients who had surgery plus adjuvant radiotherapy or chemotherapy or both. In neuroblastoma and nephroblastoma, prognosis was better in patients who had surgery plus adjuvant therapies. In hepatoblastoma, however, no advantage of adjuvant therapies was seen. As to adjuvant chemotherapy *per se*, we were not able to demonstrate its advantage or disadvantage in this study.

Neuroblastoma: Total removal of primary tumor yielded a 2-year survival rate of 58% and even a subtotal removal of the tumor showed a 2-year survival rate of 37%. Survivors were seen even in cases which had partial removal (6%) or biopsy only (15%). In Stage IVs disease, especially, 5 out of 6 cases survived.

Breakdown of the patients into stages of the disease showed that in all Stage I patients, total removal of the primary tumor was done and irrespective of adjuvant therapy or not or in the former situation, adding radiotherapy or chemotherapy, the 2-year survival rate was 100%. In the majority of Stage II patients, total removal of the tumor supplemented with chemotherapy plus radiotherapy was done and their 2-year survival rate was 67%. In Stage III patients for whom total or subtotal removal was made, adjuvant chemotherapy or radiotherapy or both were utilized in almost all patients and the 2-year survival rate was 56% for patients who had total removal and 62% in patients who had subtotal removal. However, in 19 patients who ended with partial removal or biopsy, only one patient who had chemotherapy and radiotherapy survived. In Stage IVa patients, prognosis wsa grave (4%) irrespective of the amount of the tumor removed or whether there was adjuvant therapy or not. On the contrary the 2-year survival rate of IVb disease was 30% and 2 cases each of patients who had total removal or biopsy only and one each of patients who had subtotal or partial removal survived (total 6) due to chemotherapy plus radiotherapy. However, 5 of those 6 cases were patients less than 6 months old. In Stage IVs disease, the 2-year survival rate (65%) was relatively high irrespective of total removal or biopsy only, due to adjuvant chemotherapy or radiotherapy (total: 11 survivors). However, 8 of those 11 cases were patients less 6 months old.

Primary liver cell carcinoma: A 2-year survival rate was obtained in 49% of patients who had curative surgery. On the other hand, no patients survived after relative curative surgery or biopsy only. Thus, the absolute necessity of curative removal of the tumor in achieving cure was reconfirmed. Our analysis revealed that adjuvant chemotherapy or radiotherapy was not effective in improving prognosis. However, this did not necessarily mean ineffectiveness of adjuvant therapies, since there were cases who, due to chemotherapy, had preoperative shrinkage of the tumor mass, thereby having made a curative resection possible.

Nephroblastoma: Only 11 cases were treated with surgery or surgery plus radiotherapy. The rest of 75 cases were treated with surgery plus chemotherapy or surgery plus chemotherapy and radiotherapy. The 2-year survival rate was 25% in patients treated with surgery alone, while it was over 50% in patients treated with surgery plus adjuvant

TABLE III. Method of Treatment and Prognosis

Surgery / Adjuvant therapies	Neuroblastoma — Surgery for primary tumor					Total	Primary liver cell carcinoma			Total	Nephroblastoma
	Total removal	Subtotal removal	Partial removal	Biopsy only	(−)		Curative surgery	Relative curative surgery	Biopsy only		Curative surgery
(−)	2/3		0/1	0/6	0/2	2/12 (17%)	5/9	0/5	0/6	5/20 (25%)	1/4 (25%)
Ra	3/5	1/1	0/1	1/3		5/10 (50%)	1/3			1/3 (33%)	5/7 (71%)
Ch	10/20	1/2	1/6	3/19	0/10	15/57 (26%)	8/13	0/5	0/9	8/27 (32%)	8/16 (50%)
Ra+Ch	27/45	8/24	0/9	5/31	0/7	40/116 (34%)	3/10		0/10	3/20 (15%)	29/59 (49%)
Total	42/73 (58%)	10/27 (37%)	1/17 (6%)	9/59 (15%)	0/19 (0%)	62/195 (32%)	17/35 (49%)	0/10 (0%)	0/25 (0%)	17/70 (24%)	43/86 (50%)

(Neuroblastoma Ra–Ra+Ch Total: 33%; Primary liver cell carcinoma Ra–Ra+Ch Total: 24%; Nephroblastoma Ra–Ra+Ch: 51%)

No. of survivors/all cases. 2-Year survival rate in %.

therapies. As to the method of treatment, there was a tendency as the disease progressed for the mortality to increase. In this study, no definite value of adding chemotherapy was demonstrated, however, one survivor each from Stage IV and V disease was a patient who had had adjuvant chemotherapy. After 1972, however, treatments following NWTS were commenced, and it seems that the 2-year survival rate has been increasing in recent years.

Acute Leukemia

In 4 years, namely 1957, 1962, 1967, and 1972, a total of 145 cases of acute leukemia were treated in 8 institutions in Japan and a retrospective analysis was made as to their symptoms, treatment and survival time.

Their ages ranged from 0 to 14 years, but 50% were less than 5 years old. Sixty-eight had myelogenous leukemia and 74 had lymphatic or unclassified leukemia. The rest had miscellaneous types of leukemia. All types were evenly distributed in each year. Table IV shows that the number of drugs used for each patient increased during the year. Also increasing were the remission rate and complication rate. Complications included intracranial lesion, hemorrhage, infections, and so on. The remission rate was

TABLE IV. Number of Drugs Used in Each Case

	1957	1962	1967	1972	Total
No. of cases	31	34	38	42	145
Total number of drugs used in each case					
Steroids	20	29	35	42	126
Cytotoxic drug	25	38	89	182	334
Total	45	67	124	224	460
Average for each case	1.45	1.97	3.26	5.33	3.17

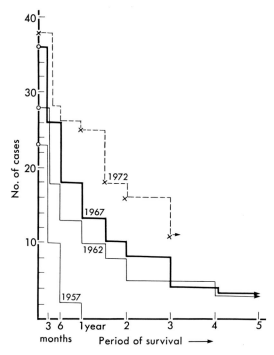

FIG. 1.　Survival curves of patients treated in each year

11.5% in 1957, 38.5% in 1962, 42% in 1957, and 88.1% in 1972. The complication rate was 1.2% in 1957, 1.2% in 1962, 1.7% in 1967, and 1.8% in 1972.

　　Figure 1 shows the survival curves of patients seen for the first time in each year. All patients who were seen in 1957 were dead within one year. In contrast, patients who visited for the first time in 1972 showed a significant improvement in survival time in comparison with patients seen in 1962 and 1967, and 11 of 42 patients lived more than 3 years. In conclusion, the survival time of acute leukemia in infancy and childhood has been prolonged remarkably in recent years, but seemingly, more drugs are necessary in achieving this, making the complication rate higher. It is important that this aspect be considered in the future.

REFERENCES

1.　Committee for Malignant Tumors, Japanese Association of Pediatric Surgeons: Staging classifications of childhood solid tumors (neuroblastoma, nephroblastoma and malignant tumors of the liver). *J. Japan. Assoc. Pediatr. Surg.*, **7**, 127–137 (1971).
2.　Committee for Childhood Malignant Tumors, Japanese Association of Pathologist: Histological classifications of nephroblastoma. *J. Japan. Assoc. Pediatr. Surg.*, **8**, 333–338 (1972).
3.　Committee for Childhood Malignant Tumors, Japanese Association of Pathologist: Histological classification of neuroblastoma. *J. Japan. Assoc. Pediatr. Surg.*, **9**, 529–535 (1973).
4.　Committee for Childhood Malignant Tumors, Japanese Association of Pathologist:

Histological classification of primary liver cell carcinoma in infancy and childhood. *J. Japan. Assoc. Pediatr. Surg.*, **10**, 142–148 (1974).

5. Committee for Malignant Tumors, Japanese Association of Pediatric Surgeons: Revisions of staging classifications of neuroblastoma, Wilms' tumor and primary liver cell carcinoma. *J. Japan. Assoc. Pediatr. Surg.*, **10**, 429–435 (1974).

CANCER STATISTICS IN JAPAN AND IN OSAKA*

Incidence, Therapy, and Survival

Isaburo Fujimoto and Aya Hanai

Osaka Cancer Registry, Department of Field Research,
*Center for Adult Diseases**

As one of the co-operative studies within the Research Group for Population-based Cancer Registration, the cancer incidence in Japan was estimated twice, in 1974 and in 1975, from the data of five population-based cancer registries: Miyagi, Kanagawa, Osaka, Tottori, and Okayama. The total population of the five prefectures was 16.1 million, or 16% of the whole population in Japan. Estimated incidence rates for all sites in Japan in 1972 were 193.6 per 100,000 population in males and 167.8 in females. The most frequent sites in males were the stomach, lung, liver, esophagus, rectum, colon, and pancreas, in that order. In females they were stomach, uterus, breast, lung, liver, colon, and rectum. The age-specific incidence rates by site and sex were presented.

The following were observed in the Osaka Cancer Registry: (1) Incidence of cancers of certain sites were changing. During 1963–1973, cancer of the stomach and uterus decreased by 20–25% and cancer of the lung, colon, and pancreas increased by more than 25%. (2) Data of 16,103 cases, who had been diagnosed in 1972–1973 in Osaka, were analyzed regarding the medical care for cancer. The proportion of cases in relation to various medical examinations, ratio of admission, and also the proportion of the type of treatment employed were calculated, by site and sex. (3) Survival rates were also presented for all cancer cases registered, by site, sex, age group, and type of treatment employed. The 5-year survival rate of cancer of all sites diagnosed during 1968–1971 was 17.6% for males and 28.1% for females.

In Japan, a national cancer morbidity survey was conducted by the Ministry of Health and Welfare (9) in four prefectures in 1959. However, the cancer incidence for the whole of Japan was not estimated from the results of this survey.

A population-based cancer registration started first in Miyagi Prefecture in 1957, followed by Aichi and Osaka 5 years later. As of 1975, cancer registration was in opera-

* Nakamichi 1-3-3, Higashinari-ku, Osaka 537, Japan (藤本伊三郎, 花井 彩).

This is a report of the Research Group for Population-based Cancer Registration. This group has been supported by a research grant from the Ministry of Health and Welfare, since 1975. Study personnel were: Isaburo Fujimoto, Aya Hanai, Akira Oshima, and Fumio Sakaue (Osaka Cancer Registry), Yasuo Anno and Takayuki Nose (Tottori Cancer Registry), Akira Takano (Miyagi Cancer Registry), Yoshio Akitani and Reiko Inoue (Kanagawa Cancer Registry), Kazuhiko Irie and Michihiro Nishida, (Hyogo Cancer Registry), Kaname Nukada (Okayama Prefectural Government), and Iwao Senoh (Kawasaki University Hospital).

tion in 16 prefectures. Besides these registries, Okayama Prefectural Government has repeated a one-year morbidity survey every 3 to 4 years. It was regrettable, however, that all these programs were carried out quite independently of each other until 1972.

In order to encourage these registration activities, 2 research groups were organized in 1972. One was supported by a research grant from the Ministry of Health and Welfare and the other of the Japan Cancer Society. Eight registries participated in the first group and 4 were the members of the second.

Six registries (Miyagi, Kanagawa, Osaka, Hyogo, Tottori, and Okayama) already had some kind of experience in incidence analysis. It was felt necessary, however, to standardize the computation procedure. In 1974, as a co-operative study within the first research group, cancer morbidity and mortality data from the 6 registries were collected and re-calculated, using uniform sheets, by the Osaka Cancer Registry (5). Thus, it became possible to compare the incidence between different registries and also to estimate the nation-wide cancer incidence.

At the expiry of the term of these two research aids in March, 1975, a new research group for cancer registration was set up under a grant from the Ministry of Health and Welfare. All population-based cancer registries joined it. Activities of the 2 former groups were handed over to the new one. The research group decided to estimate cancer incidence in Japan, using the data from participating registries, every year. In the 2nd survey in 1975, the same 6 registries presented their data. Calculation was again conducted by the Osaka Cancer Registry.

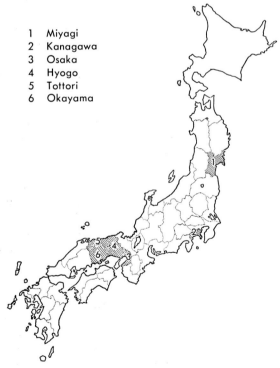

1   Miyagi
2   Kanagawa
3   Osaka
4   Hyogo
5   Tottori
6   Okayama

FIG. 1.   Location of the prefectures with population-based cancer registries that participated in the first and the second survey

This report deals with the incidence data obtained through the second co-operative surgery. Trend of cancer incidence and 5-year survival rate for cancer patients in Osaka are also observed during the period of 1963–1973.

Incidence and Treatment of Cancer in Japan

1. Participating registries in the co-operative surveys

Location of the perfectural registries who participated in the first and the second survey is shown in Fig. 1. Four are geographically close to each other.

Table I shows the survey period, the number of cancer cases found in 2 surveys, and the census population of 1970, in each prefecture. There are 59 thousand cases in the first and 40 thousand in the second survey. The total population of 6 prefectures was 21.8 million, or 21% of the whole population in Japan.

TABLE I. Survey Period, Number of Cancer Cases Observed,
and Population of Six Prefectures

Prefecture	Survey period		Number of cancer cases		Population
	1st	2nd	1st	2nd	Census of 1970
Total	—	—	59,451	39,861	21,854,309
Miyagi	1968–1971	1971–1972	11,236	6,099	1,819,223
Kanagawa	1970	1971	7,368	7,109	5,472,247
Osaka	1970–1971	1972	21,313	11,477	7,620,480
Hoygo	1971–1972	1972	13,415	6,822	4,667,928
Tottori	1969–1970	1969–1971	2,541	3,694	567,405
Okayama	1969	1973	3,578	4,660	1,707,026

2. Completeness and accuracy of the data

The proportion of the number of cases registered from death certificates only is regarded as an index of the incompleteness of cancer incidence data. Table II shows the figures among the cancer incidence of all sites in each registry. These were relatively high, probably reflecting the fact that hospital-based cancer registry or hospital medical record library is still immature in Japan. Figures in the second survey were a little smaller than those of the first. Completeness of registration improved in each registry. An artificial increase of the percentage was seen in Okayama which was caused by a modification of the computation method.

Table II also presents the proportion of the histologically confirmed cases to the registered cases with cancer reports. These ratios show the accuracy of diagnoses in reported cases. They increased in all registries except Tottori where the 2 survey periods overlapped each other. Even in the second survey, however, these ratios were lower than in many European countries and the U.S.A. (63–97% in 1959–1966) (11). This probably has many causes; the relative frequency of cancer cases of inaccessible sites, shortage of pathologists, and inadequate payment by the health insurance for a histology test.

3. Estimation of cancer incidence in Japan

Cancer incidence in Japan was estimated in the first and the second surveys. Com-

TABLE II. Completeness and Accuracy of Registry Data in the First
and Second Survey by Prefecture, All Sites

Prefecture	Male (%)		Female (%)	
	1st	2nd	1st	2nd
Proportion of cases with death certificate only[a]				
Total	35.7	31.6	31.4	27.6
Miyagi	30.7	29.5	26.1	27.6
Kanagawa	45.7	35.1	39.5	28.2
Osaka	34.9	28.1	31.4	25.6
Hyogo	62.1	50.2	54.8	45.2
Tottori	31.2	26.5	27.5	24.3
Okayama	9.5	19.9	9.2	14.5
Proprtion of histologically confirmed cases[b]				
Total	40.0	45.7	50.3	57.5
Miyagi	55.5	68.2	62.2	73.3
Kanagawa	37.5	42.7	49.6	53.0
Osaka	40.6	42.8	49.8	52.3
Hyogo	34.0	37.6	44.7	61.8
Tottori	35.1	21.9	46.6	44.0
Okayama	37.3	51.1	49.1	60.3

[a] Proportion among incidence.

[b] Proportion among reported cases.

TABLE III. Completeness and Accuracy of Five Registries' Data
by Site and Sex in the Second Survey

Site	ICD No.	Proportion of cases with death certificate only[a] (%)		Proportion of histologically confirmed cases[b] (%)	
		Male	Female	Male	Female
All sites	140–209	27.8	24.0	47.3	56.6
Esophagus	150	31.3	32.6	35.9	35.3
Stomach	151	23.7	25.2	46.2	42.0
Colon	153	21.0	28.3	51.6	52.1
Rectum	154	23.5	24.4	48.2	40.0
Liver	155, 197.8	34.8	40.2	20.6	16.9
Pancreas	157	41.2	39.6	36.1	32.5
Larynx	161	22.9	22.7	71.8	67.2
Lung	162	32.7	33.8	31.8	31.9
Breast	174	—	7.1	—	74.6
Uterus	180–182, 234.0	—	11.8	—	78.6
Bladder	188	19.5	28.2	52.9	48.3
Leukemia	204–207	38.2	36.5	38.2[c]	42.7[c]

[a,b] Described in the footnote to Table II.

[c] Cases with bone marrow puncture.

pleteness and accuracy of whole data used for the estimation in the second survey are shown in Table III.* The data from Hyogo Registry were found unsatisfactory and they were excluded.

* Cancer sites described in this report correspond to the ICD Numbers shown in Tables III and V.

The proportion of cases registered from death certificate alone was large in cancer with a higher fatality: Esophagus, liver, pancreas, lung, and blood. The proportion of cases with histological confirmation were large in cancer of accessible sites, such as the larynx, breast, and uterus.

First, the age-specific incidence rates for Japan were estimated for each site and sex by calculating the arithmetic mean of the age-specific rates from the five registries. We did not divide the total number of cancer cases by the total population of the five prefectures because, if we did so, it would obscure the characteristics of prefectures with a smaller population. Tables IV-A and IV-B show average incidence rates by age group and sex for various sites in the second survey.

At the second step, these rates were multiplied by the population of the corresponding age group for all Japan. The sum of the calculated cancer cases in each age group was divided by the total population of Japan. In this manner, the number of cases and the incidence rates in Japan were calculated, as shown in Table V. The percentage of incidence by site is also listed in the table.

Around 1972, it was calculated the cancer incidence rate for all sites in Japan was 196 per 100,000 population for males and 168 for females. The number of total cancer cases was calculated at 101,773 for males, 90,427 for females, and 192,200 for both sexes. The most prevalent was stomach cancer in both sexes. In males it was followed by lung, liver, esophagus, rectum, colon, and pancreas, in that order. In females, the second highest was uterine cancer, followed by breast, lung, liver, colon, and rectum.

To confirm the reliability of this estimated incidence, the average crude death rates of the five participating prefectures were compared with those of all Japan, in

TABLE IV-A. Age-specific Incidence Rates for All Japan in the Second Survey
(Average of Five Registries' Data) (Male)

Age	All Sites	Eso- phagus	Sto- mach	Colon	Rec- tum	Liver	Pan- creas	Lung	Bladder	Leu- kemia
All ages	198.1	7.2	89.4	6.1	7.4	14.3	5.8	22.2	5.5	4.7
0– 4	14.9	0.0	0.1	0.0	0.0	0.4	0.0	0.1	0.0	2.5
5– 9	9.9	0.0	0.0	0.0	0.0	0.4	0.0	0.1	0.0	5.0
10–14	9.8	0.0	0.6	0.1	0.0	0.1	0.0	0.0	0.0	2.4
15–19	10.4	0.0	0.5	0.1	0.0	0.3	0.0	0.0	0.0	3.7
20–24	16.2	0.0	1.5	0.5	0.4	1.1	0.1	0.7	0.0	2.6
25–29	26.1	0.4	8.4	0.7	1.9	2.2	0.0	0.5	0.3	3.3
30–34	32.1	0.2	13.3	1.5	0.3	1.7	0.4	2.0	0.6	4.0
35–39	68.4	0.9	32.5	3.0	3.9	3.3	1.3	3.7	1.0	3.4
40–44	109.2	1.2	54.0	5.6	3.4	8.1	3.1	4.6	2.2	5.0
45–49	184.9	3.1	91.6	10.2	7.6	17.9	5.6	10.2	4.3	3.8
50–54	328.5	9.4	162.9	10.5	11.0	29.6	10.8	26.2	9.7	7.5
55–59	532.8	20.4	257.9	18.5	16.7	41.2	17.9	59.7	12.4	7.3
60–64	816.5	36.3	390.9	21.0	23.0	64.0	28.1	102.4	18.9	8.9
65–69	1,164.8	51.5	522.0	30.0	46.4	78.1	37.2	156.0	30.6	8.4
70–74	1,606.5	83.2	713.6	41.6	58.8	108.6	42.5	234.7	51.5	15.0
75–79	1,846.6	109.7	813.6	68.9	65.7	127.7	59.6	253.8	67.7	6.0
80–84	1,893.4	93.5	765.5	60.3	109.6	161.9	48.9	230.7	85.3	6.3
85–	1,635.3	88.1	645.2	17.8	75.4	102.7	40.6	235.9	78.0	14.0

TABLE IV-B. Age-specific Incidence Rates for All Japan in the Second Survey
(Average of Five Registries' Data) (Female)

Age	All sites	Eso-phagus	Sto-mach	Colon	Rec-tum	Liver	Pan-creas	Lung	Breast	Uterus	Blad-der	Leu-kemia
All ages	168.8	2.8	52.8	6.6	6.7	7.4	4.9	8.1	17.2	32.7	2.0	3.2
0- 4	13.2	0.0	0.0	0.0	0.0	0.3	0.1	0.1	0.0	0.0	0.1	6.9
5- 9	6.0	0.0	0.0	0.0	0.0	0.0	0.0	0.0	0.0	0.0	0.0	2.0
10–14	9.2	0.0	0.1	0.0	0.0	0.0	0.0	0.4	0.0	0.0	0.0	3.0
15–19	10.5	0.0	0.6	0.2	0.1	0.0	0.0	0.5	0.4	0.3	0.0	2.2
20–24	15.3	0.0	3.9	0.6	0.1	0.3	0.0	0.0	0.4	0.7	0.1	3.6
25–29	26.8	0.0	8.6	0.4	0.7	0.4	0.1	0.0	3.5	4.9	0.4	1.1
30–34	52.8	0.3	15.1	0.7	1.2	1.2	1.0	1.2	9.2	11.8	0.4	2.5
35–39	104.8	0.4	29.2	3.0	4.9	0.9	2.0	1.0	18.1	32.7	0.1	2.6
40–44	167.4	0.5	41.8	2.6	5.6	2.8	2.1	4.0	37.5	56.9	0.2	2.6
45–49	241.3	0.7	60.4	8.6	7.7	5.8	3.5	6.9	48.2	79.7	0.8	2.1
50–54	284.3	3.1	74.8	8.0	10.7	7.2	5.9	11.2	43.7	86.8	4.3	4.4
55–59	409.5	4.3	132.0	15.2	11.3	14.1	10.2	24.4	42.6	91.9	2.9	3.8
60–64	534.7	10.3	167.0	21.2	19.4	28.6	20.9	28.8	46.8	91.7	7.1	4.8
65–69	645.9	15.3	211.0	27.1	27.2	41.1	23.0	42.8	40.0	90.4	12.7	7.5
70–74	843.1	20.4	311.0	42.7	37.1	55.7	32.3	64.7	35.4	101.8	12.9	4.6
75–79	1,003.5	41.9	380.0	52.9	54.6	71.1	42.2	53.9	32.9	87.7	18.4	6.0
80–84	1,016.5	40.4	410.5	57.2	51.3	70.7	41.2	63.1	38.0	67.5	16.8	3.3
85–	977.4	50.3	314.2	62.5	50.7	75.6	35.4	60.1	47.7	78.5	17.5	0.0

TABLE V. Estimated Cancer Incidence and Incidence Rates for All Japan (1972)

Site	ICD No.	Incidence		Incidence rate[a]		Proportion of incidence (%)	
		Male	Female	Male	Female	Male	Female
All sites	140–209	101,773	90,427	196.3	167.8	100.0	100.0
Buccal cavity and pharynx	140–149	1,685	859	3.3	1.6	1.7	1.0
Esophagus	150	4,064	1,626	7.8	3.0	4.0	1.8
Stomach	151	45,558	28,050	87.9	52.0	44.8	31.0
Colon	153	3,216	3,461	6.6	6.4	3.4	3.8
Rectum	154	3,670	3,460	7.1	6.4	3.6	3.8
Liver	155, 197.8	7,455	4,033	14.4	7.5	7.3	4.5
Pancreas	157	2,966	2,581	5.7	4.9	2.9	2.9
Larynx	161	1,471	225	2.8	0.4	1.4	0.2
Lung	162	11,471	4,421	22.1	8.2	11.3	4.9
Bone	170	659	648	1.3	1.2	0.7	0.7
Skin	172, 173	461	662	1.7	1.2	0.9	0.7
Breast	174	—	9,330	—	17.3	—	10.3
Uterus	180–182, 234.0	—	17,607	—	32.6	—	19.4
Ovary	183	—	2,145	—	4.0	—	2.4
Bladder	188	2,772	1,060	5.3	2.0	2.7	1.2
Leukemia	204–207	2,308	1,688	4.5	3.1	2.3	1.8

[a] Per 100,000 population.

TABLE VI. Comparison of Crude Death Rates of Malignant Neoplasms between
the Second Survey and All Japan in 1972

Site	Male			Female		
	2nd survey (A)	All Japan (B)	Difference (C)	2nd survey (A)	All Japan (B)	Differenec (C)
All sites	145.9	137.5	+ 6.1	110.7	103.9	+ 6.5
Esophagus	6.3	7.2	−12.5	2.4	2.2	+ 9.1
Stomach	61.6	58.6	+ 5.1	39.4	36.3	+ 8.5
Colon	3.6	4.0	−10.0	4.4	4.4	0
Rectum	5.1	5.2	− 1.9	4.6	4.4	+ 4.5
Liver	14.0	11.6	+20.7	7.2	6.8	+ 5.9
Pancreas	5.4	5.5	− 1.8	4.9	3.8	+28.9
Lung	19.0	17.0	+11.8	6.4	6.4	0
Breast	—	—	—	5.6	5.1	+ 9.8
Uterus	—	—	—	12.0	11.8	+ 1.7
Bladder	2.7	2.3	+17.4	1.3	1.2	+ 8.3
Leukemia	4.1	4.0	+ 2.5	2.9	3.2	− 9.4

$C = (A - B) \div B \times 100$ (%).

the vital statistics for the year 1972. They were higher in those five prefectures than in all Japan for most of the sites with the exception of the male esophagus, rectum, pancreas, and female leukemia. The difference was within the range of $\pm 13\%$ for many sites as shown in Table VI. Only a few sites showed a large difference: Male liver ($+21\%$), bladder ($+17\%$), and female pancreas ($+29\%$).

4. Comparison of cancer incidence rates between the two surveys

Table VII presents the crude incidence rates and the age-adjusted incidence rates of all Japan, estimated in the first and the second survey. The world population presented by the UICC was employed as the standard population in calculating age-adjusted incidence rates.

TABLE VII. Age-adjusted Cancer Incidence Rates in the First and the Second Survey
(Average of Five Registries' Data)

Site	Male		Female	
	1st survey	2nd survey	1st survey	2nd survey
All sites	197.1	205.2	146.7	149.5
Esophagus	8.3	8.3	2.5	2.6
Stomach	92.0	91.6	46.6	45.5
Colon	5.8	6.3	5.1	5.6
Rectum	6.5	7.4	5.6	5.6
Liver	13.6	15.1	6.6	6.6
Pancresa	5.3	6.0	3.7	4.2
Lung	19.9	23.4	6.5	7.3
Breast	0.2	0.3	14.0	15.5
Uterus	—	—	25.9	29.0
Bladder	4.9	5.7	1.9	1.7
Leukemia	4.3	4.8	2.9	3.3

In the short period, averaging 2 years, between the first and the second surveys the incidence of cancer rose for some sites and declined for others. The incidence of cancer of the colon, pancreas, lung, and breast rose and that of the stomach declined. A remarkable increase of uterine cancer was observed in Table VII. This was caused by the high incidence of only one prefecture (Okayama). In the other four prefectures incidence rates were constant or decreasing.

5. Treatment of cancer patients in Japan

In addition to the incidence rates, information was also obtained as to medical care of cancer cases. Table VIII shows the proportion of admitted patients and of surgically treated patients among the reported cases in the second survey.

The proportion of admitted cases (in-patients) was available only from two registries: Osaka and Hyogo. It was slightly higher among males than females.

The average proportion of cases treated surgically was calculated from the data of five registries other than Kanagawa. For all sites, it was markedly higher in females than males, because in females breast and uterine cancer accounted for 28% of all cases. Though not shown in the Table, it is known that medical care for cancers of several sites improved during the period between these two surveys.

TABLE VIII. Percent Admitted and Percent Treated Surgically among
Reported Cancer Cases in the Second Survey

Site	Percent admitted[a]		Percent treated surgically[b]	
	Male	Female	Male	Female
All sites	69.3	67.7	43.0	54.3
Esophagus	61.8	54.3	16.9	24.2
Stomach	77.2	69.2	57.1	56.2
Colon	72.6	76.2	77.4	74.7
Rectum	88.0	74.5	65.7	60.8
Liver	53.8	67.1	10.7	9.9
Pancreas	64.6	61.1	46.4	41.5
Lung	56.8	59.1	14.0	19.3
Breast	—	83.3	—	81.7
Uterus	—	69.9	—	56.4
Bladder	50.0	—	44.3	—
Leukemia	58.3	50.7	3.4	1.2

[a] Data obtained from Osaka and Hyogo.
[b] Data obtained from Miyagi, Osaka, Hyogo, Tottori, and Okayama.

Cancer Statistics in Osaka

1. Trends of cancer incidence in Osaka

In Osaka, prefecture-wide cancer registration has been in operation since December, 1962, under co-operation of the Osaka Medical Association, the Health Department of Osaka Prefectural Government, and the Center for Adult Diseases, Osaka (4, 6, 7). The central registry has been set up in the Center for Adult Diseases. About 130 thousand cancer cases have been registered in the past 12 years.

TABLE IX. Age-adjusted Incidence Rates by Survey Period, 1963-1973, Osaka

Site	Male				Female			
	1963–1965	1966–1968	1969–1971	1972–1973	1963–1965	1966–1968	1969–1971	1971–1972
All sites	216.1	211.1	204.6	204.3	160.1	152.0	143.8	140.2
Esophagus	10.9	9.8	9.2	9.1	3.5	3.5	3.0	2.5
Stomach	109.2	101.2	92.1	85.3	52.8	49.8	45.9	41.7
Colon	4.3	5.4	6.2	6.3	3.5	4.6	5.1	5.7
Rectum	7.1	6.1	6.9	6.8	4.7	4.9	4.7	3.9
Liver	17.1	16.2	15.4	17.4	9.0	7.3	6.9	6.7
Pancreas	4.6	5.6	5.5	5.8	2.4	2.9	3.1	3.3
Lung	19.1	20.7	22.9	26.2	6.3	6.4	6.8	7.9
Breast	—	—	—	—	11.0	11.0	11.9	13.7
Uterus	—	—	—	—	39.8	33.8	29.6	28.7
Bladder	—	5.1	5.1	5.6	—	2.0	1.5	1.6
Leukemia	—	3.6	4.0	3.7	—	2.5	3.1	2.9

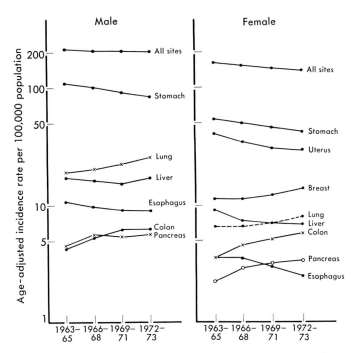

FIG. 2. Trends in age-adjusted incidence rates by site, 1963–73, Osaka

Osaka Prefecture had a population of 7,620,480 at the 1970 census. The capital city, Osaka, is surrounded by 30 satellite cities, 11 towns, and 2 villages. There are 5 medical schools, 454 hospitals, and 6,006 private clinics; 10,923 physicians were working in 1974.

Table IX presents the age-adjusted cancer incidence rates for selected sites in each triennial period since the inception of the registry. These trends are illustrated graphically in Fig. 2.

TABLE X. Proportion of Increase or Decrease of Age-adjusted Incidence Rates
and Death Rates, 1963-1973, Osaka

Site	Trend of incidence rate[a] (%)		Trend of death rate[a] (%)	
	Male	Female	Male	Female
All sites	− 5.5	−12.4	− 3.2	− 3.9
Esophagus	−16.5	−28.6	−13.8	−24.1
Stomach	−21.9	−21.0	−20.8	−17.7
Colon	+46.5	+62.9	+30.3	+55.6
Rectum	− 4.2	−14.0	+ 5.7	− 8.3
Liver	+ 1.8	−25.6	*	*
Pancreas	+26.1	+37.5	+21.4	+50.0
Lung	+37.1	+25.4	+46.7	+40.0
Breast	—	+24.5	—	+54.1
Uterus	—	−27.9	—	−25.3
Bladder	*	*	*	*
Leukemia	*	*	+72.4	0

[a] [(rate in 1972–1973) − (rate in 1963–1965)] ÷ (rate in 1963–1965) × 100 (%).
* Incalculable.

Table X shows the degree of increase and decrease in cancer morbidity and mortality, by site and sex. The difference in age-adjusted incidence rate for each site between the two periods, 1972–1973 and 1963–1965, was divided by the rate in 1963–1965. In the same way, the ratio was calculated for mortality, using the data of vital statistics in Osaka.

A decrease was seen in cancers of the stomach and esophagus in both sexes, and

TABLE XI. Medical Care for Cancer

	All sites	Esophagus	Stomach
Number of cases with report	16,103	501	5,836
Proportion of cases received (%)			
1) X-ray	71.6	86.2	82.2
2) Endoscopy	28.8	35.3	44.2
3) Cytology	28.3	16.7	15.2
4) Histology	52.4	37.3	40.8
5) 3) and/or 4)	60.3	41.7	44.8
Proportion of cases admitted (%)	75.2	73.0	70.8
Proportion of treatment (%)			
1) Surgery (S) only	21.7	12.7	28.2
2) Radiation (R) only	4.8	9.9	0.2
3) Chemotherapy (C) only	13.4	11.3	11.4
4) S and R	6.7	13.5	0.2
5) S and C	16.5	6.5	25.0
6) R and C	2.8	5.7	0.2
7) S, R, and C	4.3	8.9	0.5
8) Others and unkown	24.3	25.9	28.2

in the uterus and liver in females. An increase was seen in cancers of the lung, colon, and pancreas in both sexes, and in the breast in females.

2. Medical care of cancer patients in Osaka

Table XI presents figures related to the medical care of cancer patients who had been diagnosed in 1972–1973 and reported to the registry.

The upper half of the Table shows the proportion of patients who were examined by X-ray, endoscopy, cytology, and histology. Although it is not shown in the Tables, all the percentages were increasing annually. For example, the proportion of endoscopic examination for stomach cancer was 29.2% in 1966–1968 and rose to 44.2% in 1972–1973. The proportion of microscopically confirmed cases, shown as "cytology and/or histology," was 47.8% in 1966–1968 and 60.3% in 1972–1973, for all sites.

The proportion of cancer patients who were admitted to hospitals was, as shown in Table XI, in the range of 70–90%.

The lower half of Table XI presents percent distribution of the types of medical treatment conducted for cancer patients. Treatment was classified as "surgery only," "radiation only," "chemotherapy only," "any combination of these methods," and "others and unknown." The proportion of cases who have received surgical operation with or without other treatment was 53.9% for cancer of the stomach, 60.6% for uterus, but only 16.2% for lung and 10.1% for liver. Radiation with or without chemotherapy was conducted for 20.9% of uterine cancer cases.

3. Five-year survival rates of cancer patients in Osaka

Since a hospital-based cancer registry has not been common in Japan, information about survival and prognosis of registered cases is not available, except for those from death certificates, in most population-based cancer registries. Thus, 5-year survival

Cases in 1972–1973, Both Sexes, Osaka

Colon	Rectum	Liver	Pancreas	Lung	Breast	Uterus
579	512	914	345	1,482	888	1,881
81.5	63.4	63.5	77.6	92.5	69.2	28.1
22.1	43.7	11.7	21.1	19.9	1.2	30.6
12.7	11.7	23.6	17.9	64.3	7.4	80.1
53.1	52.3	22.8	36.5	37.9	81.8	86.8
55.6	54.6	37.8	43.4	71.1	82.8	92.3
83.9	80.2	75.2	82.6	72.9	88.4	78.0
38.5	36.9	5.7	28.4	4.8	21.8	27.4
0.3	0.5	0.3	0.5	6.1	2.8	16.4
4.8	5.6	27.1	12.7	30.8	1.5	2.3
1.5	3.7	0.2	0.8	2.3	22.0	24.9
33.8	23.2	4.2	17.9	5.0	22.7	3.4
0.1	0.5	0.9	0.0	7.8	0.7	4.5
1.7	3.1	0.0	0.2	4.1	19.8	4.9
13.8	19.3	53.3	32.1	34.3	7.0	12.4

rates for cancer cases in the general population have never been reported. The Commission on Cancer of the American College of Surgeons (1) concluded that the end results should be most valuable for measuring the quality of cancer programs. We decided, accordingly, to try to calculate survival rates based on the data available in our registry.

Confirmation of death of the registered cases was made only by collating them with death certificates mentioning cancer from Osaka residents. All the unmatched cases were regarded as alive. However, these unmatched cases must include a certain proportion of cases who had left Osaka and then died and cases who had died from other causes than cancer.

In order to estimate the degree of this bias, a follow-up study was made on a sample of 829 cancer cases. These were the cases diagnosed at the Center for Adult Diseases in 1968. It become clear that if the calculation of survival was based on the collation with death certificate alone, then the magnitude of overestimation would be about 11% (for cancer of all sites).

Another difficulty was that 25–28% of the cancer incidence was registered from death certificates alone, and their lengths of survival were not known. These cases

TABLE XII.　Five-year Relative Survival Rates for Selected Sites, Osaka and U.S.A.

| | | 5-Year survival rate (%) | | | Number of cases observed | | |
| | | Japan | U.S.A. | | Japan | U.S.A. | |
Site	Sex	Osaka 1965–1968	California 1965–1969	Connecticut 1955–1963	Osaka 1965–1968	California 1965–1969	Connecticut 1955–1963
All sites	Male	17.6	32.3	—	20,207	29,232	—
	Female	28.1	48.0	—	17,913	30,172	—
Stomach	Male	20.0	12.1	11.2	9,760	1,111	1,899
	Female	16.6	13.1	15.4	5,715	754	1,135
Colon	Male	25.0	46.4	38.3	377	2,017	2,984
	Female	22.1	47.8	43.3	336	2,474	3,470
Rectum	Male	24.1	38.6	34.8	622	1,286	1,911
	Female	20.1	45.6	39.1	565	1,147	1,571
Pancreas	Male	5.8	1.8	2.7	524	789	899
	Female	4.6	3.3	3.1	320	664	581
Lung	Male	7.9	7.8	7.9	1,868	5,934	4,184
	Female	10.1	12.3	9.8	698	1,690	735
Breast	Female	58.4	65.7	59.5	1,382	7,634	7,659
Cervix uteri	Female	64.0	58.4	60.6	2,181	2,806	1,903
Corpus uteri	Female	69.5	71.5	72.9	133	2,263	1,734
Bladder	Male	34.8	52.9	60.0	432	1,812	2,079
	Female	20.5	54.5	65.8	202	664	717
Leukemia	Male	5.3	11.1	2.7[a] 5.2[b]	439	994	209[a] 347[b]
	Female	3.3	13.8	3.0[a] 27.2[b]	336	754	176[a] 226[b]

[a] Acute leukemia.
[b] Chronic leukemia.

were regarded as dead within 5 years after diagnosis. (From the analysis of fatal cases for all sites, whose survival periods were known to us, it was known that 97.4% died within 5 years.)

Cancer cases diagnosed in 1965–1968, totalling 38,120 primary cancers of all sites, were thus followed until December, 1973. The 5-year relative survival rate was computed by Cutler's method (2). The expected survival rate was employed from those figures calculated by Koike (8) from the data of the life table in Japan in 1965–1974.

In Table XII, 5-year relative survival rates in Osaka are shown together with the corresponding rates in Connecticut (3) and California (10) in the U.S.A. The survey period is longer in Connecticut than in other places. In Osaka, patients with cancer of the stomach (female), lung (both sexes), breast (female), and uterus had almost the same survival as those in the other two registries. For stomach cancer, male patients had a more favorable survival rate in Osaka than in the other two. On the contrary, cases with cancer of the colon and rectum showed lower survival rates in Osaka.

Table XIII presents 5-year relative survival rates for four selected sites by the treatment method. The figures were omitted from the table where the number of observed cases was less than 50. In all 4 sites the rate was highest in the group treated by surgery only.

Table XIV shows 5-year relative survival rates for four selected sites by age group. In general, the younger age group had a more favourable survival.

TABLE XIII. Five-year Relative Survival Sates by Type of Treatment, 1965–1968, Osaka

Type of treatment	Stomach		Lung		Breast	Uterus
	Male	Female	Male	Female	Female	Female
5-Year relative survival rate (%)						
Surgery (S) only	30.8	28.3	20.5	25.3	76.6	73.7
Radiation (R) only	—	—	15.2	—	—	59.9
Chemotherapy (C) only	9.1	7.4	6.1	4.3	—	14.0
S and R	—	—	—	—	73.0	70.7
S and C	28.7	23.8	—	—	72.6	46.1
R and C	—	—	3.4	—	—	19.1
S, R, and C	—	—	—	—	63.2	55.1
Others and unknown	14.5	12.0	7.0	9.8	35.2	31.2
Number of cases observed						
Surgery only	2,419	1,244	100	34	462	1,074
Radiation only	15	5	71	14	9	242
Chemotherapy only	451	270	263	104	13	75
S and R	22	8	23	7	158	733
S and C	939	481	37	10	114	55
R and C	10	5	71	15	5	57
S, R, and C	28	9	25	7	91	97
Others and unknown	5,876	3,693	1,278	507	530	1,850

Five-year survival rate was not presented if the number of cases observed was less than 49.

TABLE XIV. Five-year Relative Survival Rates by Age Group, 1965-1968, Osaka

Age	Stomach		Lung		Breast	Uterus
	Male	Female	Male	Female	Female	Female
5-Year relative survival rate (%)						
–39	27.2	16.8	16.9	—	63.2	67.2
40-69	21.3	18.6	8.4	9.2	58.1	50.2
70–	11.0	9.9	4.5	11.5	48.0	29.5
Number of cases observed						
–39	562	545	60	39	265	683
40-69	6,899	3,612	1,289	466	986	3,069
70–	2,299	1,558	519	193	131	431

DISCUSSION

The cancer incidence in Japan was estimated from the data of 5 population-based cancer registries. The number of cancer patients in 1972 reached 192,200 for all sites. The most frequent cancer sites in both sexes were the stomach, uterus, lung, liver, breast, rectum, and colon, in that order. This co-operative survey has been continuing with participation of 14 registries.

Changes in cancer incidence in Osaka were remarkable, although the observation period was rather limited. It is necessary to ascertain whether such changes have been occurring in other prefectures as well. At the same time, it will be essential to start an epidemiological study on the causes of these changes.

Survival rates were also computed from the data of the Osaka Cancer Registry. This is the first data of its kind in Japan for population-based cancer incidence. The 5-year survival rate of cancer cases of all sites was 17.6% for males and 28.1% for females. For stomach cancer it was 20.0% in males and 16.6% in females, and for cancer of the cervix uteri it was 64.0%.

In 1977, one year after contributing this report, the Osaka Cancer Registry modified the follow-up method. Now, all death certificates are used for collation with cancer reports, instead of death certificates mentioning cancer. The magnitude of overestimating the survival rate becomes smaller; 6% of survival rate for cancer cases for all sites.

REFERENCES

1. Copeland, M. M. and Cline, J. W. Commission on Cancer of the American College of Surgeons. *Cancer*, **20**, 596–600 (1967).
2. Cutler, S. J. Computation of survival rates. *Natl. Cancer Inst. Monogr.*, **15**, 381–385 (1963).
3. Eisenberg, H., Sullivan, P. D., and Connelly, R. R. "Cancer in Connecticut, Survival Experience, 1935–1962." Connecticut State Dept. Health, Hartford, pp. 93–114 (1968).
4. Fujimoto, I. Role of cancer registration. *Gan-no-Rinsho* (*Cancer Clinic*), **21**, 969–975 (1975) (in Japanese).
5. Fujimoto, I., Hanai, A., Sakaue, F., Takano, A., Inoue, R., Nishida, M., Nose, T., and

Senoh, I. Cancer incidence and medical care in Japan, 1970. *Kosei-no-Shihyo* (*J. Health Welfare*), **22** (4), 3–15 (1975) (in Japanese).

6. Hanai, A., Fujimoto, I., Oshima, A., Dodo, H., Satani, H., Nakamura, Y., and Nakatani, H. Cancer incidence in Osaka, Japan, 1963–66. *Annu. Rep. Center Adult Dis.*, **9**, 1–18 (1969).

7. Hanai, A., Sakaue, F., and Fujimoto, I. Computerized cancer registration collation system—quantitative study on record linkage. *Annu. Rep. Center Adult Dis.*, **13**, 1–15 (1973).

8. Koike, A. and Tashiro, S. Expected survival rates, 1965–70. *Kosei-no-Shihyo* (*J. Health Welfare*), **23** (3), 14–27 (1967) (in Japanese).

9. Ministry of Health and Welfare. "The Second National Cancer Survey, 1960," Tokyo, pp. 1–61 (1962) (in Japanese).

10. Personal communication from California Tumor Registry.

11. UICC. "Cancer Incidence in Five Continents," ed. by R. Doll, C. Muir, and J. Waterhouse, International Union Against Cancer, Geneva, Vol. II, pp. 384–385 (1970).

SUBJECT INDEX